PSYCHIATRIC/
MENTAL HEALTH
NURSING
REVIEW

ARCO NURSING REVIEW SERIES

PSYCHIATRIC/ MENTAL HEALTH NURSING REVIEW

Janet Ahalt Rodgers, Ph.D., R.N.
Associate Professor and Coordinator
of Psychiatric Nursing
Department of Nursing
Herbert H. Lehman College
The City University of New York
Bronx, NY

Weslee Neary McGovern, M.A., R.N.
Instructor of Psychiatric Nursing
Department of Nursing
Herbert H. Lehman College
The City University of New York
Bronx, NY

Arco Publishing Company, Inc.
New York

Second Printing, 1977

Published by Arco Publishing Company, Inc.
219 Park Avenue South, New York, NY 10003

Library of Congress Catalog Card Number 73-86238
ISBN 0-668-03374-6

Printed in the United States of America

Library of Congress Cataloging in Publication Data

Rodgers, Janet Ahalt.
  Psychiatric/mental health nursing review.

  1. Psychiatric nursing—Examination, questions, etc.
I. McGovern, Weslee Neary, joint author. II. Title.
[DNLM: 1. Psychiatric nursing—Examination questions.
WY18 R691p]

RC440.R65   610.73'68   73-86238
ISBN 0-668-03374-6

For Terry
who has the patience of Job

For my husband, Gene
and
my sons, Tiger, Chris, and Andy

Contents

Preface

The primary purpose of this book is to assist nursing students in reviewing for examinations in psychiatric nursing. We have written it with the realization that nurses with different educational preparation will be reading it, and we believe that it will offer assistance on these different levels. A secondary purpose of the book is to serve as a tool for nurses wishing to continue their education and up-date their knowledge of this field.

The type of questions presented are modeled after standardized examinations; they are of the multiple choice and matching type. The situational type format has been extensively utilized in order to test application of knowledge through simulated experiences from nursing practice. The answer to each question has been individually referenced and explanations incorporate the theoretical principles that the authors considered.

Acknowledgements

Many of our colleagues in the Department of Nursing at Herbert H. Lehman College have contributed ideas for test questions. We thank them for the ideas and for their tolerance of our groans and mutterings. We also thank those students who willingly offered to take selected portions of the test and give us feedback.

Our special gratitude goes to the three secretaries who typed the manuscript—Mrs. Santa Pompei, Mrs. Joyce Clancy and Miss Margaret Doody. In particular, we want to express our affection to Mrs. Pompei for her organization and patience from the beginning to end and to Mrs. Clancy for her lively sense of humor.

References

Below is a numbered list of reference books pertaining to the material in this book.

On the last line of each test item, at the right hand side there appears a number combination that identifies the reference source and the page or pages where the information relating to the question and the correct answer may be found. The first number refers to the textbook in the list and the second number refers to the page of that textbook.

For example: (33: 78–79) is a reference to the thirty-third book in the list, pages 78–79 of Sutterley and Donnelly's *Perspectives in Human Development*.

Where volume number is indicated, the reference reads, for example: (6:II:23) which is a reference to the sixth book in the list, volume two, page 23 of Arieti's (et al) *American Handbook of Psychiatry*.

1. Aguilera, D., and Messick, J. M. *Crisis Intervention.* Saint Louis: The C.V. Mosby Company, 1974.
2. Almeida, E.M., and Chapman, A.H. *The Interpersonal Basis of Psychiatric Nursing.* New York: G.P. Putnam's Sons, 1972.
3. American Nurses Association. *Statement on Psychiatric Nursing Practice.* Kansas City: American Nurses Association, 1967.
4. American Psychiatric Association. *A Psychiatric Glossary.* Washington: American Psychiatric Association Publications Office, 1969.
5. Anderson, R.E. and Carter, I. E. *Human Behavior in the Social Environment.* Chicago: Aldine Publishing Co., 1974.
6. Arieti, S. (ed). *American Handbook of Psychiatry,* Vol. I, II, and III. New York: Basic Books, Inc. 1974.
7. *Blakiston's Gould Medical Dictionary.* New York: McGraw-Hill, Inc., 1972.
8. Boyd, R. and Oakes, C.G. (eds.) *Foundations of Practical Gerontology.* 2nd Ed. Columbia: University of South Carolina Press, 1973.
9. Burd, S.F., and Marshall, M.A. *Some Clinical Approaches to Psychiatric Nursing.* New York: The Macmillan Company, 1963.
10. Burgess, A.C., and Lazare, A. *Psychiatric Nursing in the Hospital and the Community.* Englewood Cliffs: Prentice-Hall, Inc., 1973.
11. Burkhalter, P.K. *Nursing Care of the Alcoholic and Drug Abuser.* New York: McGraw-Hill Book Co., 1975.
12. Cadoret, R.J. and King, L.J. *Psychiatry In Primary Care.* Saint Louis: The C.V. Mosby, Co., 1974.
13. Evans, F. *Psychosocial Nursing.* New York: MacMillan Publishing Company, Inc., 1971.
14. Fagin, C.M., (ed). *Nursing in Child Psychiatry.* Saint Louis: The C.V. Mosby Company, 1972.
15. Huey, F.L. (ed). *Psychiatric Nursing 1946 to 1974.* New York: The American Journal of Nursing Company, 1975.
16. Irving, S. *Basic Psychiatric Nursing.* Philadelphia: W.B. Saunders Company, 1973.
17. Joint Commission on Mental Illness and Health. Report of the Commission, *Action for Mental Health.* New York: Basic Books, Inc., 1961.
18. Kalkman, M.E., and Davis, A.J. (eds). *New Dimensions in Mental Health-Psychiatric Nursing.* New York: McGraw-Hill Book Company, 1974.

19. Klein, D.C. *Community Dynamics and Mental Health.* New York: John Wiley & Sons, 1968.
20. Kolb, L.C. *Modern Clinical Psychiatry.* Philadelphia: W.B. Saunders Company, 1973.
21. Kyes, J.J. and Hofling, C.K. *Basic Psychiatric Concepts in Nursing.* Philadelphia: J.B. Lippincott Company, 1974.
22. LeBow, M.D. *Behavior Modification.* Englewood Cliffs: Prentice-Hall, Inc., 1973.
23. Loomis, M.E. and Horsley, J.A. *Interpersonal Change.* New York: McGraw-Hill, Inc., 1974.
24. Lugo, J.O., and Hershey, G.L. *Human Development.* New York: Macmillan Publishing Company, Inc., 1974.
25. MacKinnon, R.A., and Michels, R. *The Psychiatric Interview* in *Clinical Practice.* Philadelphia: W.B. Saunders Company, 1971.
26. Manfreda, M.L. *Psychiatric Nursing.* Philadelphia: F.A. Davis Company, 1973.
27. Mereness, D. (ed). *Psychiatric Nursing.* Vol. I and Vol. II. Dubuque: Wm. C. Brown Company Publishers, 1971.
28. Mereness, D.A., and Taylor, C.M. *Essentials of Psychiatric Nursing.* Saint Louis: The C.V. Mosby Co., 1974.
29. Mitchell, P.H. *Concepts Basic to Nursing.* New York: McGraw-Hill, Inc., 1973.
30. Morgan, A.J., and Moreno, J.W. *The Practice of Mental Health Nursing: A Community Approach.* Philadelphia: J.B. Lippincott Company, 1973.
31. Resnik, H.L.P. and Ruben, H.L. (eds.). *Emergency Psychiatric Care.* Bowie, Md.: The Charles Press Publishers, Inc. 1975.
32. Rosenbaum, C.P. and Beebe, J.E. *Psychiatric Treatment.* New York: McGraw Hill, Inc., 1975.
33. Sutterley, D.C., and Donnelly, G.F. *Perspectives in Human Development.* Philadelphia: J.B. Lippincott Company, 1973.
34. Travelbee, J. *Intervention in Psychiatric Nursing.* Philadelphia: F.A. Davis Company, 1969.

CHAPTER I

Epidemiology and History: An Overview of the Field

INTRODUCTION

The primary purpose of this chapter is to review the major epidemiological factors of mental health and illness as well as the historical development of mental health care.

It is the belief of the authors that in order to understand the current forces at work in psychiatric care and be able to intelligently predict future trends, it is imperative for the nurse practitioner to have a sense of the historical development of both psychiatry and psychiatric nursing. The causative factors, that is, the incidence, distribution, prevalence, and control of mental disorders, are also important in order to develop a theoretical framework that provides a basis for prevention and treatment. Therefore, this chapter will utilize both multiple choice and matching questions to enable the readers to evaluate their present knowledge of the areas of the epidemiology of mental health and illness and the history and trends in mental health care.

A. Epidemiology of Mental Illness

Directions: For each of the following multiple choice questions, select the ONE most appropriate answer.

1. Which of the following is the best indicator of good mental health?

   A. development of insight
   B. ability to function effectively
   C. capacity to develop an object relationship
   D. freedom from anxiety   (13:61–2)

2. Mental illness is generally agreed upon to be due to

   A. a thought disorder
   B. a genetic factor
   C. an interpersonal problem
   D. none of the above   (20:123–26)

3. All of the following describe a mentally healthy person *except*

   A. he has a capacity to invest in others
   B. he lacks emotional conflicts
   C. he is spontaneous in work and social relations
   D. he has a high energy level   (20:88)

4. All of the following are common *misconceptions* about mental illness *except*

   A. masturbation is a frequent precursor of mental illness
   B. a psychosis can be precipitated by a real or imagined loss
   C. a person who is truly religious will never become mentally ill
   D. a highly intelligent person who comes from the upper middle class is unlikely to become mentally ill   (20:360–61)

1

5. Sex is an important variable in mental illness in that

    a. the admission rate to hospitals for mental disorders is 6 men to 5 women
    b. more women than men actually reside in public mental hospitals
    c. organic psychoses are more common in men than women
    d. both involutional depression and schizophrenia are more common among women than men

    A. a and c
    B. b only
    C. b and d
    D. all of the above   (20:128–29)

6. Which of the following is most accurate in terms of assessing the variable of sex in influencing mental illness?

    A. there are usually more beds for male patients than female patients
    B. there are usually more beds for female patients than male patients
    C. the significance of sex as a vulnerability to psychiatric disorder is difficult to assess
    D. none of the above   (10:316–17)

7. Which of the following life events ranks highest in stress potential according to the Social Readjustment Rating Scale?

    A. change in financial state
    B. divorce
    C. death of spouse
    D. personal injury or illness   (32:12–13)

8. Holmes and Rahe predict that a major depression or physical illness is likely within a year if a person obtains a score on the Social Adjustment Rating Scale higher than

    A. 120
    B. 150
    C. 235
    D. 300   (32:12)

9. In several studies of mental illness in children, it has been found that aggressive patterns of behavior are more frequent in children of

    A. blue collar workers
    B. unskilled workers
    C. skilled workers
    D. professional persons   (18:491)

10. Which of the following statements regarding post partum disorders are true?

    a. postpartum psychoses are statistically rare
    b. postpartum disorders are considered a separate diagnostic category
    c. half of postpartum psychoses are schizophrenic episodes
    d. organic brain deliriums are frequent in postpartum disorders

    A. a and b
    B. b and c
    C. a and c
    D. a, b, c, and d   (2:359)

11. The incidence of psychoses is greatest among individuals

    A. 0 to 3 years of age
    B. 8 to 12 years of age
    C. 35 to 40 years of age
    D. 60 to 80 years of age   (20:128)

12. The number of people in a large population who could be diagnosed schizophrenic

    A. differs from culture to culture from 0 to 5%
    B. has increased since 1900 to about 5%
    C. remains fairly constant at about 1%
    D. has decreased since the 1950's to about 0.1%   (20:312)

13. The most susceptible age group for the onset of schizophrenia is from

    A. 5 to 15 years
    B. 15 to 20 years
    C. 15 to 45 years
    D. 35 to 50 years   (20:312)

14. Which of the following statements about schizophrenia are accurate?

    a. 50% of the resident population in state mental hospitals are diagnosed as schizophrenic

    b. 25% of the resident population in state mental hospitals are diagnosed as schizophrenic

    c. schizophrenia is a major mental health problem in modern society

    d. schizophrenia is chiefly a thought disorder

    A. a and b
    B. a, b, and c
    C. a, c, and d
    D. b, c, and d   (20:308–12; 10:228)

15. In 1964, what percentage of first admissions to state mental hospitals in the U.S. were diagnosed as psychoneurotic?

    A. 4.6%
    B. 25%
    C. 11.3%
    D. 40%   (18:338)

16. According to the official statistics, the rate of suicide is highest in which country?

    A. United States
    B. Northern Ireland
    C. West Germany
    D. Italy   (32:27)

17. Suicide is most common in the United States in the age group of

    A. 15 to 24
    B. 25 to 34
    C. 55 to 64
    D. 85 and older   (32:27)

18. Which of the following individuals falls in the lower risk category for suicidal potential?

    A. a 55 year old male alcoholic
    B. a 35 year old divorced physician
    C. a white Protestant male lawyer
    D. a black Catholic taxi driver   (32:26)

19. Which of the following predisposing psychiatric conditions is the most predictive of suicide?

    A. drug or alcohol problems
    B. depression
    C. manic-depressive illness
    D. past suicidal history   (32:30–1)

20. Predisposing personality styles for suicide are the

    A. impulsive
    B. compulsive
    C. risk-taking
    D. all of the above   (32:29–30)

21. A high homicide rate is positively correlated with

    A. very low socioeconomic class
    B. lack of a high school education
    C. the tendency to carry hand guns
    D. all of the above   (32:65)

22. The therapist should recognize that the most important key to controlling homicide is the patient's control of

    A. aggression
    B. impulsivity
    C. narcissism
    D. masochism   (32:75–80)

23. Factors commonly present in the personal childhood histories of those who later commit murder include

    a. severe emotional deprivation or overt rejection
    b. parental seduction
    c. exposure to brutality and extreme violence
    d. fire-setting
    e. cruelty to animals or children

    A. a and b
    B. a and c
    C. a, c, d, and e
    D. all of the above   (32:66)

24. All of the following statements concerning murder and females are true *except*

    A. females kill males more often than they do females
    B. black females murder 3 times as frequently as white males
    C. butcher knives are the preferred weapon of females
    D. females are most commonly slain by firearms   (32:64–5)

25. Which of the following is *true?*

    The majority of murders in this country are

        a. committed by blacks
        b. committed on blacks
        c. committed by males
        d. committed on males

    A. a and b
    B. a and c
    C. a, b, and c
    D. all of the above   (32:64–5)

26. All of the following statements regarding the incidence of alcoholism are true *except*

    A. there are between 9 and 10 million alcoholics in the U.S.
    B. men have a higher rate of alcoholism than women
    C. alcoholism is a major problem among teenagers
    D. alcoholism ranks fourth as a major health problem in the U.S.   (11:6)

27. The incidence of alcoholism is thought to be

    A. two times greater among men than women
    B. five times greater among men than women
    C. two times greater among women than men
    D. five times greater among women than men   (11:6)

28. Which of the following groups accounts for the highest percentage of problem drinkers?

    A. skid row type

B. inner city dweller
C. blue collar worker
D. upper class executive   (32:116)

Questions 29 to 33 refer to the Hollingshead-Redlich study of the epidemiology of mental illness.

29. The study was carried out in

    A. New York City
    B. Los Angeles
    C. New Haven
    D. San Francisco   (20:131)

30. In arriving at an Index of Social Position (indicator for social class), Hollingshead and Redlich used all of the following criteria *except* the

    A. residential address of a household
    B. occupational position of the head of the household
    C. years of school the head of the household had completed
    D. current salary earned by the head of the household   (6:vol.III:182–83)

31. The study mentioned in the previous question indicates a positive correlation between

    A. neuroses and the middle class
    B. neuroses and the lower class
    C. psychoses and the upper class
    D. psychoses and the lower class
                        (6:vol.III:182)

32. The diagnostic category most common in the highest socioeconomic groups was

    A. paranoid schizophrenia
    B. phobia
    C. obsessive-compulsive disorder
    D. manic-depressive psychosis   (20:131)

33. One of the most important findings of this study was

    A. Class I, the highest socioeconomic class, was composed of the community's business and professional leaders

B. Class V, the lowest socioeconomic class, contributed by far the largest percentage of identified patients

C. the family members of those in Class II, the second highest socioeconomic class, are "joiners"

D. Class IV included families with the most broken homes (1:45–7)

Questions 34 to 36 refer to the Midtown Manhattan Study.

The Midtown Manhattan Study is an example of an epidemiological study which was carried out in the late 1950's.

34. The study was carried out by

A. interview method
B. questionnaires
C. use of hospital and agency records
D. phone contacts (20:127)

35. A major finding of the study was that

A. 60% of the respondents were found to have *some* psychiatric illness
B. approximately 1 in every 5 persons was considered "mentally impaired"
C. approximately 1 in every 10 persons was considered to be "mentally impaired"
D. 30% of the respondents were found to have *some* psychiatric illness (20:127)

36. Chronological age as a variable indicated that

A. there was an increase in poor mental health with increasing age
B. there was a decrease in poor mental health with increasing age
C. the factor of age was not a significant variable in one's mental health status
D. the researchers of the study did not analyze the variable of years of age (10:316)

B. History and Trends in Mental Health Care

Directions: For each of the following multiple choice questions, select the ONE most appropriate answer.

37. A physician who has been described as the first psychiatrist is

A. Sigmund Freud
B. Hippocrates
C. Cornelius Agrippa
D. Johann Weyer (20:4)

38. Exorcism was practiced extensively in

A. Ancient Greek Civilization
B. The Middle Ages
C. sixteenth century England
D. sixteenth century United States (20:4)

39. Which of the following men helped release the mentally ill from their chains and dungeons and change society's attitudes toward the mentally ill?

A. Vincenzo Chiaruggi
B. Phillipp Pinel
C. Benjamin Rush
D. all of the above (16:71)

40. The city of Gheel in Belgium is known

a. for having the first organized colony plan for caring for the mentally ill
b. as the birthplace of Sigmund Freud
c. for utilizing the concept of family treatment within the community structure
d. as the capitol of Belgium

A. a
B. b and c
C. a and c
D. d (28:323–24)

41. Which of the following reasons does Ullman propose for the high recovery rates of psychiatric patients in the U.S. during the early nineteenth century?

   a. patients were expected to be healthy
   b. the superintendent, his family, and staff provided models of health
   c. the medical model of care was initiated
   d. immigrants were the predominant occupants of the patient role

   A. a
   B. b and d
   C. a and b
   D. c and d   (6:vol.III:30)

42. The first psychiatrist to describe and classify psychiatric disorders in a systematic way was

   A. Sigmund Freud
   B. Emil Kraepelin
   C. Eugen Bleuler
   D. Adolf Meyer   (20:4)

43. The Swiss psychiatrist who elaborated Kraepelin's concept of dementia praecox and expanded it into a theory of schizophrenia was

   A. Maxwell Jones
   B. Adolf Meyer
   C. Sandor Rado
   D. Eugen Bleuler   (20:309–11)

44. The physician known as the Father of American Psychiatry was

   A. Philippe Pinel
   B. Benjamin Rush
   C. Emil Kraepelin
   D. Sigmund Freud   (28:329–30)

Directions: Each group of numbered words or phrases is followed by a list of lettered statements. MATCH the lettered statement most closely associated with the numbered word or phrase.

Questions 45 to 52

45. William Tuke   (26:41)
46. Amariah Brigham   (26:43)
47. Samuel B. Woodward   (26:42)
48. Pythagoras   (26:32)
49. Hippocrates   (26:33)
50. Plato   (26:33)
51. Asclepiades   (26:33)
52. Juvenal   (26:31)

   A. Descriptions of depressive and neurotic symptoms
   B. Psychosomatic view
   C. Father of Psychiatry
   D. *American Journal of Insanity*
   E. York Retreat
   F. American Psychiatric Association
   G. Thought mental illness was caused in the brain
   H. Senile dementia

Directions: For each of the following multiple choice questions, select the ONE most appropriate answer.

53. Dorothea Lynde Dix, a pioneer crusader for reform in the treatment of mental illness,

   A. was a retired school teacher who worked with prisoners in Massachusetts jails
   B. became superintendent of Female Nurses in the Army in 1861
   C. helped to found St. Elizabeth's Hospital in Washington, D.C.
   D. all of the above   (28:325)

54. Clifford Beers, a former mental patient, was

   a. the author of *A Mind That Found Itself*
   b. a graduate of Yale University
   c. the founder of the National Committee for Mental Hygiene

d. instrumental in initiating child guidance centers, prison psychiatry, and vocational guidance

A. a
B. a and c
C. a, c, and d
D. all of the above   (28:326)

55. The physician who first attempted to cure many diseases including hysteria by his technique of "animal magnetism," later called hypnotism, was

A. Anton Mesmer
B. Jean Martin Charcot
C. Pierre Janet
D. Josef Breuer   (20:7)

56. One of Freud's most significant discoveries is considered to be the

A. origin of hypnosis
B. "transference phenomena"
C. treatment of schizophrenia
D. understanding of the psychosis(1:11–14)

57. All of the following statements about Sigmund Freud are true *except* that he

A. was originally trained as a neurologist
B. first developed the psychotherapeutic technique of "cathartic hypnosis"
C. was the founder of what is known as psychoanalysis
D. was only interested in the psychological as opposed to the physiological aspects of human behavior   (20:8–9)

58. The psychiatrist first interested in the psychobiological approach to mental illness or the longitudinal study of a patient's life was

A. Carl Jung
B. Benjamin Rush
C. Jacob Moreno
D. Adolf Meyer   (20:11)

59. Word-association tests were first used in psychotherapy by

A. Carl Jung
B. Sigmund Freud
C. Kurt Lewin
D. Karen Horney   (12:238)

60. The psychiatrist known for studying the relationship of artistic creations, mythological themes, and religion to dreams, phantasies and neuroses is

A. Sigmund Freud
B. Jean Charcot
C. Adolf Meyer
D. Carl Jung   (20:10–11)

61. All of the following statements about Carl Jung are true *except* that he

A. believed that the unconscious is made up of two sources, the "personal unconscious" and the "collective unconscious"
B. was the first to suggest a psychological approach to the study of dementia praecox
C. was the first to recognize that neurotic symptoms have "meaning"
D. developed the concept of introversion-extroversion   (20:8–11)

62. The theory of the inferiority complex is attributed to

A. Freud
B. Jung
C. Adler
D. Reich   (4:21)

63. Alfred Adler, an early student and associate of Freud who later came to disagree with Freud's emphasis on infantile sexuality, believed that

A. a child's drive to self assertion, domination, and superiority were more important than the sexual drive
B. because of a sense of inferiority, a will to power is stimulated
C. each individual has his own unique goals and unique manner of achieving them
D. all of the above   (20:9–10)

64. The term "Oedipus Complex" was first introduced by

    A. Harlow
    B. Erikson
    C. Freud
    D. Bleuler   (20:53)

Directions: Match the numbered term with the letter of the therapist most closely associated with it. Letters (therapists) may be used more than once or not at all.

Questions 65 to 73

65. Logotherapy   (12:253)
66. Free association   (12:236–37)
67. Analytical psychology   (12:238)
68. Therapeutic dialectics   (12:251)
69. Existentialism   (12:253)
70. Life space   (12:245–46)
71. Inferiority complex   (12:239)
72. Will and counter-will   (12:241)
73. Nondirective technique   (12:247)

    A. Carl Rogers
    B. Otto Rank
    C. Alfred Adler
    D. Victor Frankel
    E. B. F. Skinner
    F. Sigmund Freud
    G. Kurt Lewin
    H. Carl Jung
    I. Jergen Ruesch

Questions 74 to 82

74. Instrumental or operant conditioning
                                  (12:248)
75. Respondent or classical conditioning
                                  (12:247)
76. Transference neurosis   (12:237)
77. Gestalt therapy   (12:245–46)
78. Birth trauma   (12:241)
79. Introversion-extraversion   (20:11)
80. Psychobiology   (12:243)
81. Striving for power   (12:239–40)
82. Collective unconscious   (12:238)

    A. Sigmund Freud
    B. Ivan Pavlov

C. Otto Rank
D. Carl Jung
E. B. F. Skinner
F. Alfred Adler
G. Kurt Lewin
H. Adolf Meyer
I. Anton Mesmer

Directions: For each of the following multiple choice questions, select the ONE most appropriate answer.

83. Adolf Meyer who played a prominent role in the development of dynamic psychiatry in the United States was

    A. older than Freud but had similar interests in the medical sciences
    B. primarily known for his "psychobiological" approach
    C. concerned with the short term history of clients
    D. of the belief that all people were basically alike   (20:11)

84. Which of the following men proposed constellations of morphologic, physiologic, and psychologic traits?

    a. Galin
    b. Sheldon
    c. Jung
    d. Kretschmer

    A. a and d
    B. b and c
    C. a and c
    D. a, b, and d   (4:25)

85. Harry Stack Sullivan is best known for his development of

    A. intrapsychic theory
    B. interpersonal theory
    C. communications theory
    D. psychobiological theory   (20:11)

86. The founder of modern psychosurgery is

    A. Moniz
    B. Bini
    C. Watts
    D. Freeman   (21:413)

87. Franz Kallmann is best known for his

    A. contribution to communication theory
    B. research on manic-depressive illness
    C. writing on general systems theory
    D. research on schizophrenia involving twin studies   (20:125–26)

Directions: Match the following numbered items with the most appropriate lettered items.

Questions 88 to 92

88. Applied term psychoneurosis to hysteria
                                     (20:8)
89. Introduced the term hypnotism   (20:8)
90. Introduced Freudian psychoanalysis in America   (2:532)
91. Introduced Freudian psychoanalysis in England   (2:532)
92. Developed the first intelligence test   (2:533)

    A. A. A. Brill
    B. H. M. Bernheim
    C. Ernest Jones
    D. Simon and Binet
    E. James Braid

Directions: For each of the following multiple choice questions, select the ONE most appropriate answer.

93. Goffman considers mental hospitals similar to

        a. jails
        b. military units
        c. monasteries
        d. convents

    A. a
    B. a and b
    C. c and d
    D. a, b, c, and d   (6:III:30–31)

94. Carl Rogers is best known for his

    A. client-centered therapy
    B. behavior therapy
    C. will therapy
    D. gestalt therapy   (12:246)

95. According to Berne, transactions involve the fluctuating, interchanging ego states in each person of

    A. parent
    B. child
    C. adult
    D. all of the above   (12:252)

96. Eric Berne is best known for his use of

    A. learning theory
    B. systems theory
    C. game theory
    D. communication theory   (12:251–52)

97. Ronald D. Laing is a British psychoanalyst who believes that schizophrenia is

    A. a reaction to an impossible life situation
    B. not an illness, but rather an experience into madness and return
    C. the result of cultural pressure on the schizophrenic to be "normal" or like others
    D. all of the above   (18:331)

98. The founder of Synanon is

    A. Lewis Yablonsky
    B. Marty Mann
    C. Charles Dederich
    D. Father Daniel Egan   (18:408)

Directions: Match the following numbered items with the most appropriate lettered item.

Questions 99 to 103

99.	Kanner	(6:II:89)
100.	Bender	(6:II:88)
101.	Bowlby	(6:II:253)
102.	Spitz	(6:II:110)
103.	Coles	(18:55)

A. Anaclitic depression
B. Cultural influences
C. Growth disturbance
D. Abandonment depression
E. Early infantile autism

Questions 104 to 109

104.	Grief Work	(1:2–6)
105.	Ego Psychology	(1:2–6)
106.	Eight Stages of Psychosocial Growth and Development	(1:2–6)
107.	Psychoanalysis	(1:2–6)
108.	Preventive Mental Health	(1:2–6)
109.	Adaptational Psychotherapy	(1:2–6)

A. Heinz Hartmann
B. Sigmund Freud
C. Sandor Rado
D. Erik Erikson
E. Erich Lindemann
F. Gerald Caplan

Directions: For each of the following multiple choice questions, select the ONE most appropriate answer.

110. The basic tenets of the philosophy of a therapeutic community (Jones) are

    a. the current social behavior of the patient is the focus
    b. the patient is an active participant in his own therapy and that of other patients
    c. increased communication between staff and patients decreases social distance
    d. psychodynamic insights of personality and psychopathology are de-emphasized and work therapy is emphasized

A. a
B. a and b
C. d
D. all of the above   (10:316)

Questions 111 to 113 are based on recommendations to Congress by the Joint Commission on Mental Illness and Health in its 1961 landmark report.

111. Any construction of new state psychiatric hospitals should be limited to no more than how many beds?

A. 500
B. 750
C. 1000
D. 1750   (17:XVI)

112. The Commission also recommended which of the following actions regarding treatment facilities?

A. a fully staffed, full-time mental health clinic should be available to each 50,000 of population
B. every community general hospital of 100 or more beds should provide a psychiatric unit or psychiatric beds
C. existing state mental hospitals housing 1000 or more patients should not admit even one more patient
D. all of the above   (17:XIV–XV)

113. Secondary prevention, the detection of beginning signs and symptoms of mental illness and their relief, should be provided in the community by

    a. mental health counselors, eg., clergymen, family physicians, teachers, etc.
    b. mental health consultants, eg., psychologists, nurses, social workers, etc.
    c. pediatricians
    d. resident schools for emotionally disturbed children

A. a and b
B. b
C. b and c
D. a, b, c, and d   (17:XII–XIII)

114. The Community Mental Health Centers Act of 1963, an outgrowth of the Commission's Report, had a revolutionary impact on psychiatric nursing by

  a. requiring that a course in psychiatric nursing be taught in every undergraduate nursing program
  b. forcing the nurse to learn to participate as a coequal with other members of the psychiatric health care team
  c. encouraging the nurse to leave the security of her well-defined roles in a bureaucratic hospital system for ill-defined functions in a loosely structured mental health center
  d. demanding a higher level of accountability because of the concept that the same therapist should provide and/or be responsible for the total treatment of the patient

  A. a
  B. a and c
  C. b and c
  D. b c, and d   (18:19–22)

115. The act mandated that a community mental health center must be accessible to the community it serves. Which of the following are included in the minimum of five basic services necessary?

  a. inpatient treatment
  b. outpatient treatment
  c. diagnostic services
  d. emergency services on a 24 hour basis

  A. a and b
  B. a, b, and d
  C. b and c
  D. a, b, c, and d   (30:193)

116. A center must serve a specific area with a population of between

  A. 10,000 and 25,000
  B. 25,000 and 50,000
  C. 50,000 and 100,000
  D. 75,000 and 200,000   (30:193)

117. The term used to designate the geographic boundaries of a community mental health center is

  A. health area
  B. region
  C. district
  D. catchment area   (30:194)

118. The World Health Organization has recommended several guidelines for establishing and developing suicide prevention services. These include

  a. local emergency medical services
  b. psychiatric consultation
  c. emergency psychiatric services
  d. follow-up psychiatric care

  A. a and c
  B. a, b, and c
  C. b and c
  D. a, b, c, and d   (6:III:759)

119. The Joint Commission on Mental Health of Children studied young people from ages

  A. birth to twenty-one
  B. birth to twenty-five
  C. birth to eighteen
  D. birth to sixteen   (18:101)

120. The Joint Commission on Child Mental Health recommended

  a. initiation of programs for the prevention of mental illness
  b. program planning based on the development model
  c. program planning based on the medical model
  d. initiation of programs of treatment of mental illness

  A. a and b
  B. c and d
  C. a, c, and d
  D. a, b, and d   (18:59)

121. Which of the following organizations places emphasis on preventive aspects of mental disorders in children?

    A. American Psychoanalytic Association
    B. The Group for the Advancement of Psychiatry
    C. The American Orthopsychiatric Association
    D. The American Psychiatric Association
    (4:67)

122. The official list of disease categories of the World Health Organization is known as the

    A. *Diagnostic and Statistical Manual-II*
    B. *Index Medicus*
    C. *International Classification of Diseases*
    D. *International Manual of Nervous Disorders*
    (4:50)

123. The Center for Studies of Schizophrenia is

    A. a private foundation
    B. a federal agency
    C. a professional association
    D. an international agency
    (13:318)

124. Two alcoholic detoxification centers have been funded as demonstration projects by the

    A. U.S. Department of Justice
    B. National Commission on Alcoholism
    C. National Institute of Mental Health
    D. U.S. Public Health Department
    (13:337)

125. Which of the following organizations was the first to be dedicated to the scientific study of suicide, on a nationwide basis?

    A. the Center for Studies of Suicide Prevention
    B. the American Association of Suicidology
    C. the Public Health Department
    D. the Samaritans
    (13:271)

126. All of the following professions are products of the twentieth century *except*

    A. psychiatric social work
    B. psychiatric nursing
    C. occupational therapy
    D. recreational therapy
    (2:533–35)

127. *The Diagnostic and Statistical Manual of Mental Disorders* is utilized for making a

    A. descriptive diagnosis
    B. psychodynamic diagnosis
    C. treatment plan
    D. assessment of the client's problems
    (2:91–2)

128. Linda Richards is best known as the

    A. author of the first psychiatric nursing textbook
    B. first graduate psychiatric nurse in the United States
    C. publisher and editor of *Perspectives in Psychiatric Care*
    D. first graduate of the Cadet Nursing Program
    (18:5)

129. Hildegard Peplau is a psychiatric nursing leader known for

    a. publishing the first textbook in psychiatric nursing, *Nursing Mental Diseases*
    b. publishing the classic, *Interpersonal Relationships in Nursing*
    c. organizing and systematizing scientific knowledge so that it might be applied, tested, and integrated into the practice of psychiatric nursing
    d. having served as an expert teacher and director of the graduate programs at Teachers College, Columbia University, and Rutgers University
    e. serving as the President of the American Nurses Association from 1970–1972

    A. a and c
    B. b
    C. b and d
    D. b, c, d, and e
    (28:326)

130. Probably the single most important event influencing the course of psychiatric nursing was

    A. the fact that many of the early diploma programs in nursing were established in psychiatric hospitals
    B. the expansion of psychiatric services in V.A. Hospitals following World War II
    C. the development of a National Institute of Mental Health in 1946 which provided funds for undergraduate and graduate psychiatric nursing programs
    D. the passage of the Community Mental Health Centers Act in 1963   (18:10–11)

131. All of the following statements about psychiatric nursing education are true *except*

    A. McLean Hospital in Massachusetts offered the first "training school" for psychiatric nurses in 1882
    B. Dorothea Lynde Dix was the first American graduate psychiatric nurse
    C. The National Mental Health Act (1946) allotted large amounts of money to the development of psychiatric nursing programs in universities at both undergraduate and graduate levels
    D. Psychiatric-Mental Health Integration Grants began in 1956 and were funded through N.I.M.H.   (18:5)

132. The reason that nurses were initially slow to make use of Freud's psychoanalytic theory was that

    A. Freud was anti-women and most nurses are women
    B. Freud's concepts lacked a psychodynamic base
    C. Freud was interested only in patients with chronic schizophrenic symptoms
    D. the classical practice of psychoanalysis provided no treatment role for the psychiatric nurse   (18:7–8)

133. The psychiatric nurse first responsible for demonstrating that changes can occur as a result of nursing intervention in a nurse-patient relationship is

    A. Gwen Tudor Will
    B. Hildegard Peplau
    C. Jane Schmahl Cattell
    D. Ida Jean Orlando   (18:17)

134. The psychiatric nurse clinician/teacher best known for her intensive anaclitic work (developing and utilizing an intensive symbiotic relationship) with schizophrenic patients is

    A. Marguerite Sechehaye
    B. Theresa Muller
    C. June Mellow
    D. Hildegard Peplau   (15:6)

135. Which of the following nurses have attempted to define the role of the psychiatric nurse?

    a. Hildegard Peplau
    b. Claire M. Fagin
    c. Loretta Ford
    d. Martha Rogers

    A. a
    B. a and b
    C. b and d
    D. c and d   (27:I:127–34, 155–65)

136. According to Peplau, the emphasis in psychiatric nursing is on

    A. the managerial role
    B. mother surrogate role
    C. socializing agent role
    D. counseling role   (27:I:131)

137. The role of clinical specialist in psychiatric nursing is that of

    a. milieu therapist
    b. individual psychotherapist
    c. group therapist
    d. family therapist

    A. a only
    B. a and c
    C. b, c, and d
    D. all of the above   (3:14–19)

138. A psychiatric nurse is officially defined as

    A. a registered nurse who works in a psychiatric hospital or other psychiatric setting

    B. a registered nurse holding a master's degree from a university graduate program with clinical specialization in psychiatric nursing

    C. a registered nurse working in any type of psychiatric mental health setting who holds a baccalaureate degree in nursing

    D. a practicing registered nurse who is concerned with the mental health needs of clients in any type of health related facility   (3:14)

Directions: Match the numbered nursing texts with the letter of the nurse author most closely associated with it.

Questions 139 to 143

139. *Nurse-Patient Relationships in Psychiatry*
                                              (15:1)
140. *Interpersonal Relations in Nursing*   (15:2)
141. *The Dynamic Nurse-Patient Relationship*
                                              (15:5)
142. *Determinants of the Nurse-Patient Relationship*   (15:6)
143. *The Group Approach in Nursing Practice*
                                              (15:19)

    A. Ida Jean Orlando
    B. Gwen Marram
    C. Gertrud Ujhely
    D. Hildegard Peplau
    E. Helena Render

Chapter I: Answers and Explanations

1. **B.** A mentally healthy individual is one who meets the situational requirements of life and therefore, adapts, adjusts, and problem-solves effectively. One may have intellectual insight into one's behavior but still not be able to modify the behavior. A mentally healthy person is able to develop *healthy* object relationships. Everyone experiences anxiety but one's flexibility and competence in coping with stressful situations is the important factor.

2. **D.** Mental disorders may stem from genetic and constitutional factors, lack of ego development and failure of ego functioning, interpersonal difficulties, as well as toxic agents. There is no one etiological factor in mental illness.

3. **B.** No one is without emotional conflicts. However, the mentally healthy individual is able to respond flexibly in the face of stress, and to accept his limitations realistically.

4. **B.** Loss of an important person, role, physical attractiveness, etc., are all stresses severe enough to cause a psychosis in a vulnerable individual. The loss does not have to be physical or actual to be experienced as real.

5. **D.** More men than women are admitted to mental hospitals. However, because of the greater longevity of women, there are more females residing in public mental hospitals. Psychoses due to organic problems are more common in men than women. Manic-depressive psychoses, involutional melancholia, and psychoses with somatic disease are more frequent in women as does appear to be the diagnosis of schizophrenia.

6. **C.** Accurate data is hard to obtain because of problems in reporting. Hospital beds for males and females are generally comparable in number but admission rates vary. Many people feel that sociocultural aspects of the male and female roles have a strong influence on who is actually hospitalized.

7. **C.** The life events that lead to crisis have been studied by Holmes and Rahe. They rank the life event with greatest stress potential as being death of a spouse, with divorce falling second.

8. **D.** Each of the 43 items on the scale is ranked and assigned a mean value in terms of stress potential. A score of higher than 300 suggests a major depression or physical illness within a year.

9. **B.** The most characteristic clinical description of children of unskilled workers included such terms as overt hostility, impulsivity, paranoid reaction, affective disturbance, and withdrawal.

10. **C.** Postpartum psychoses occur about once in every thousand births. Half of postpartum psychoses are schizophrenic episodes and most of the remaining ones are either depressive or manic states.

11. **D.** Psychoses are rare until adolescence when their incidence rises sharply and continue to show a definite trend with the advance of age. Since one-half of the U.S. population lives past 65, the incidence of senile and arteriosclerotic mental disease is high.

12. **C.** Calculations made from various epidemiological surveys give the morbidity risk for the syndrome as 1%.

13. **C.** The syndrome is customarily recognized in persons from 15 to 45 years of age.

14. **C.** Not only is schizophrenia one of the most complex problems in psychiatry, but statistically, half the population in many mental hospitals is diagnosed as schizophrenic. There is disordered thinking.

15. **C.** The admission rate of psychoneurotics had gradually increased from 1950 to the point 11.3% in 1964.

16. **C.** West Germany, Austria and Hungary have official suicide rates above 20.0 per 100,000, and West Berlin 41.3 per 100,000.

17. **D.** Suicide increases, for the most part, with age, indicating the fallacy of the serenity of old age.

18. **D.** Blacks and Orientals tend to have a lower suicidal risk potential than whites and American Indians; Jews and Catholics tend to have lower than Protestants, and noncompetitive and/or low demand for interpersonal giving occupations have lower than competitive and/or demanding of interpersonal giving occupations.

19. **D.** The history of a previous suicide attempt is the single most important prognosticator of suicidal potential.

20. **D.** Individuals who cannot control impulses and those who enjoy taking gambles are both predisposed to suicide. Likewise, compulsive personalities (high-achieving and perfectionistic) are inflexible and have difficulty in adjusting to changing circumstances. The compulsive personality is predisposed to involutional depression and may for a short time become acutely suicidal.

21. **D.** In contrast to suicide, homicide is primarily a problem of the lowest socioeconomic classes and of areas where most persons did not reach high school. Although Detroit has the highest rate of any U.S. city, the highest rate in the country for nonurban areas is in the rural south (an area where whites are more likely to carry hand guns).

22. **B.** The key to controlling homicide is control of impulsivity. The therapist should take the necessary steps to help the patient separate the thought of homicide from the act and stand squarely against impulsive emotional discharge.

23. **D.** The personal background of the eventual murderer suggests considerable disequilibrium within the family and within himself. All five factors have been found by Menninger and Modlin to be commonly present.

24. **D.** A woman killing a woman is extremely rare. A woman is most commonly slain by her husband or other close friend during a beating in the bedroom.

25. **D.** The black murder rate is 16 to 17 times that of the white rate; 66% of the urban murders are between blacks and in 62% of all murders, men kill men.

26. **C.** Dependence on alcohol is extremely rare in persons under the age of twenty. Serious drinking under the age of 20 years is, however, currently on the increase.

27. **B.** At least one alcoholic in every five is a woman.

28. **C.** According to Kissin, the population of the problem drinker is "completely heterogeneous," ranging from the skid row type (less than 5%) through the inner city dweller (20%), the blue collar worker (40%), the middle class citizen (30%), to the upper class executive (more than 5%).

29. **C.** Hollingshead and Redlich, two professors at Yale, carried out their study in New Haven, Connecticut.

30. **D.** The two-factor index used to determine social position was based on (1) areas of residence, (2) occupations and level of educational achievement.

31. **D.** These two researchers found more psychotics and fewer neurotics in the lower classes than in the upper classes.

32. **C.** Obsessive-compulsive disorders were found to be most common in the highest socioeconomic groups and oedipal conflicts in the middle group.

33. **B.** Class V—those with the poorest education, jobs, and housing—also had more brittle family ties. Unable to pay for counseling or extensive psychotherapy, they sought help only as a last resort. Frequently they had repeated admissions to hospitals and often ended up dying there.

34. **B.** Rates of reported psychological disorders obtained in the Midtown Study were collected through replies to questionnaires.

35. **B.** Although 81.5% of the respondents were judged to be "less than well," only 23.4% were placed in the "impaired group."

36. **A.** Researchers found that there was an increase in poor mental health with age by decades. For example, the 50 to 59 year group indicated 15% well and 31% impaired, as compared to 24% well and 15% impaired in the 20 to 29 age group.

37. **D.** Johann Weyer was a physician who worked openly against the belief of supernatural possession as the cause of mental phenomena. He is described as the first psychiatrist.

38. **B.** With the decline of the Roman Empire and throughout the Dark Ages of Western man, there occurred a revival of demonology. Throughout the Middle Ages there were tortuous excorcisms with disagreement from only a few solitary individuals.

39. **D.** Chiaruggi (1759-1820) in Italy, Pinel (1745-1826) in France, and Rush (1745-1813) in the U.S. emphasized the humane treatment of the mentally ill.

40. **C.** In the fifteenth century, pilgrimages to Gheel from every part of the civilized world were organized for the mentally sick. It became the natural thing over the years for the inhabitants to accept these pilgrims into their homes. In 1851, the Belgian government took charge of this colony of mental patients which continues to exist to the present day.

41. **C.** In the era of moral treatment, patients were taught to behave like integrated, healthy non-patients by the attitudes and behavior of staff.

42. **B.** Following a long series of observations by brilliant clinicians in Europe, Emil Kraepelin (1856–1926) gave to psychiatry the first comprehensive description of what he believed were entities of mental disease.

43. **D.** Bleuler (1857-1939) introduced the term schizophrenia in 1911 thus supplanting the term dementia praecox.

44. **B.** Benjamin Rush (1745-1813), who is known as the father of American psychiatry, began work at the Pennsylvania Hospital in 1783.

45. **E.** William Tuke established York Retreat in 1796.

46. **D.** Amariah Brigham founded the *American Journal of Insanity,* now known as the *American Journal of Psychiatry.*

47. **F.** Samuel Woodward conceived the idea for an organization of medical superintendents which became the A.P.A.

48. **G.** Pythagoras is credited with being the first to regard mental disorder as an illness of the brain.

49. **A.** Hippocrates recognized a relationship between elation and depression. He recorded symptoms of pressures in the head and chest, symptoms of digestive complaints, and worry.

50. **B.** Plato believed that the mind and body are inseparable and that mental illness can result from bodily or moral disturbance.

51. **C.** Asclepiades used baths and diets for curing psychiatric ills. He condemned mechanical restraints.

52. **H.** Juvenal described the symptoms of memory loss as he spoke of senile dementia.

53. **D.** Dix, a 40-year-old school teacher, aroused the public conscience and effected reforms in mental health that shook the world.

54. **D.** The emphasis on prevention and recognition of early stages of mental illness was not made until Clifford Beers, an energetic, enthusiastic ex-mental patient, became active in the movement.

55. **A.** Anton Mesmer, a Viennese outcast, stirred a furor in Paris in the late 1700's with his use of what he called "animal magnetism." Although his success was short-lived, his technique was picked up and came to be known as mesmerism.

56. **B.** Freud worked primarily with neurotic individuals. The reliving of the neurotic past in a present relationship with the therapist is known as transference neurosis.

57. **D.** Originally a neurologist, Freud then turned his attention to the psychoneuroses and collaborated with Breuer in the use of hypnotism. The founder of psychoanalysis had his original education in medicine and always considered the physiological aspects of a person's condition.

58. **D.** Slightly younger than Freud but with a similar interest in the basic sciences, Meyer insisted that multiple biological, psychological, and social forces contribute to the growth and determination of personality.

59. **A.** The patient is asked to say immediately what word comes to mind when a given stimulus word is spoken to him.

60. **D.** Carl Jung greatly stressed symbology and religion in his study of the collective or racial unconscious.

61. **C.** Josef Breuer, an early associate of Freud's, was probably the first to recognize that neurotic symptoms have "meaning" in relation to the patient's previous life.

62. **C.** Adler theorized that feelings of inferiority stemmed from real or imagined physical or social inadequacies and caused anxiety or other adverse reactions.

63. **D.** Basically, Adler, an early student and associate of Freud, came to believe in the "masculine protest" and "individual psychology."

64. **C.** Sigmund Freud coined the term "Oedipus Complex" to describe the interaction that occurs during the phallic stage. This involves the child's attraction to the parent of the opposite sex accompanied by jealousy and hostility toward the parent of the same sex.

65. **D.** Frankl, a Viennese psychiatrist, was interned in a Nazi concentration camp and later developed an existential approach to psychotherapy which he called logotherapy.

66. **F.** Essential to the psychoanalytic technique developed by Freud is the use of free association. The patient is admonished to relate everything that passes through his mind even if he thinks it embarrassing, irrelevant, or nonsensical. Following every thought that comes to mind leads to the uncovering of memory gaps which have arisen through repression of psychologically painful material.

67. **H.** Jung, a Swiss psychiatrist, participated in Freud's early group of psychoanalysts in Vienna. In 1912, after much soul searching, Jung broke with Freud and began to develop his own philosophy, analytical psychology.

68. **I.** Jergen Ruesch has written extensively on communication analysis, particularly in conceptualizing the psychotherapeutic process. Some of the important techniques of his therapeutic dialetics include: pinpointing, documentation, translation, amplification, and confrontation.

69. **D.** Victor Frankel is an existentialist. Existentialism involves the analysis of being and focuses on the importance of human choice or decision.

70. **G.** Kurt Lewin is a well known gestalt psychologist who believes that only as a member of a group does an individual personality develop. Life space includes the individual and the psychological environment as it exists for him.

71. **C.** Alfred Adler, a Viennese physician, believed that even though every child feels inferior to some degree, if some part of his body is abnormal and/or if his childhood environment is unfavorable, he develops abnormal feelings of inferiority—the inferiority complex—and his unconscious goal becomes the unrealistic one of complete superiority.

72. **B.** Otto Rank believed will is comparable to the ego of other psychologies. The counterwill or ability to say "no" to others and to one's own impulses he felt was the nucleus of personality.

73. **A.** Carl Rogers is famous for his nondirective therapy. The counselor's comments are not interpretative but rather, reflect back to the client what the latter has said, sometimes restating the client's remarks but never passing judgment on them.

74. **E.** Instrumental conditioning, the conditioning of operant behavior, has been studied extensively by the Harvard psychologist, B.F. Skinner.

75. **B.** Classical or respondent conditioning was developed in the late nineteenth century by Pavlov, the Russian physician and physiologist, who experimented with a normal dog being presented with food.

76. **A.** Freud found that in order for an analysis to be successful, an analysis of the transference was necessary.

77. **G.** Gestalt therapists emphasize perception and feeling, and their relation to life's problems rather than intellectual explanations. They help the patient focus on alternative explanations of events (perception) and alternative choices of action (behavior).

78. **C.** Rank developed the concept of the birth trauma. With the separation from the mother at birth, the feeling of wholeness is lost. In every subsequent separation from important people, Rank believes one sees in the other person the mother who bore him and deserted him.

79. **D.** Among Jung's many contributions was the development of the concept of the extravert-introvert types of personality.

80. **H.** Adolf Meyer's approach to individuals' problem behavior, psychobiology, emphasized the importance of genetic, physiological, sociological, and interpersonal factors in the total development of personality.

81. **F.** Unlike sex (as in the Freudian scheme), Adler felt that in our culture, masculinity has come to be associated with power and strength and feminity with subservience and weakness. He believed the will to power develops as a response to the universal inferiority feelings in children.

82. **D.** Jung emphasized the collective unconscious, the repository of archetypes or symbolic figures common to all mankind.

83. **B.** Although slightly younger than Freud, Adolf Meyer shared Freud's interest in the basic sciences of neurology, neuroanatomy, and pathology. He insisted that multiple biological, psychological and social forces contribute to the growth and determination, of personality and emphasized the comprehensive study of the life history of the patient.

84. **D.** Galin proposed the sanguine, melancholic, choleric, and phlegmatic types. Kretschmer identified the pyknic, asthenic, athletic, and dysplastic types. Sheldon proposed the ectomorphic, mesomorphic, and endomorphic types.

85. **B.** Sullivan emphasized the communicative interchanges between the growing infant and his parents as the means of specifying the dynamic evolution of human behavior.

86. **A.** The founder of modern psychosurgery is Egas Moniz, a Portuguese neurosurgeon and neurophysiologist, who first published his work in 1936.

87. **D.** Kallmann found that the average expectancy in any group not characterized by blood relationship to a schizophrenic is 0.85% but that the children of one schizophrenic parent have a probability of developing the disease which is 19 times that of the general population. Children of two schizophrenic parents had a rate of 80 times that of average. In identical twins of such parents in which one twin is schizophrenic, the occurrence of schizophrenia in the second twin is 85.8%.

88. **B.** Hyppolyte-Marie Bernheim was probably the first to apply the term psychoneurosis to hysteria and similar states.

89. **E.** The English surgeon, James Braid, provided a descriptive formulation of mesmerism and introduced the term, hypnotism.

90. **A.** A. A. Brill (1874-1948) introduced Freudian psychoanalysis in America.

91. **C.** Ernest Jones (1879-1958) introduced Freudian psychoanalysis in England.

92. **D.** The first intelligence test was introduced in France in 1905 by Simon and Binet.

93. **D.** Goffman has included the mental hospital in his category of "total institutions" in which the normally divided areas of living, such as working, playing, sleeping, and eating, are carried out together in one place under the guidance of an overall master plan. All of the examples are total institutions.

94. **A.** The clinical psychologist, Carl Rogers, extended psychotherapy beyond the specific problems of psychiatric patients and provided counseling about life problems to clients who are not psychiatrically ill.

95. **D.** Continuously shifting parental, childish, or adult behaviors in each person interact with the continuously shifting Parent, Adult or Child of the other person or persons in a transaction.

96. **C.** Game theory involves mathematical analysis of a conflict situation which assumes that the participants are rational beings, capable of calculating the risks necessary to maximize their own gains and minimize their own losses. Eric Berne uses this approach in his transactional analysis.

97. **D.** Laing, the British psychoanalyst defines the term schizophrenia in a very broad context and believes that it is a label that some people pin on others under certain social circumstances.

98. **C.** Charles Dederich, a former alcoholic, is the founder of Synanon.

99. **E.** Leo Kanner differentiated infantile autism from schizophrenia on the basis of onset history, course, and familial background.

100. **C.** Lauretta Bender emphasized the central significance of disturbances in growth.

101. **D.** John Bowlby described the stage of (1) protest and wish for reunion (2) despair and (3) detachment if the mother was not replaced.

102. **A.** Rene Spitz described anaclitic depressions.

103. **B.** Robert Coles has studied American black children and the effects of environment on physical, mental and emotional health.

104. **E.** In his study of bereavement reactions among the survivors of those killed in the 1943 Coconut Grove nightclub fire, Lindemann described both grief and abnormally prolonged reactions to the loss of a significant person.

105. **A.** Heinz Hartmann was an early and influential ego analyst.

106. **D.** Erikson, who further developed theories of ego psychology, perceived eight stages of psychosocial development spanning the entire life cycle of man and involving specific developmental tasks that must be solved in each phase.

107. **B.** Sigmund Freud is well known for originating the treatment technique of psychoanalysis.

108. **F.** Caplan's first community-wide program of mental health, the Wellesley Project, was established in 1946 by he and Lindemann in the Harvard area. He has written a great deal about preventive mental health and the importance of crisis periods in individual and group development.

109. **C.** Rado saw human behavior as being based on the dynamic principle of motivation and adaptation. His development of the concept of adaptational psychodynamics provided a new approach to the unconscious, as well as new goals and techniques of therapy.

110. **D.** Jones views the nurse's role as a tripartite one—authoritarian, social, and therapeutic. In the therapeutic role, nurses do not work in a one-to-one relationship with the patient, but rather encourage and support him in his various therapeutic activities, including his therapeutic relationship with his psychiatrist.

111. **C.** The report recommends that no further state hospitals of more than 1000 beds should be built, and not one patient should be added to any existing mental hospital already housing 1000 or more patients.

112. **D.** The Joint Commission in its recommendations included all three areas.

113. **D.** In order to carry out secondary prevention, in the absence of fully trained psychiatrists, clinical psychologists, psychiatric social workers, and psychiatric nurses, such counseling should be done by persons with some psychological orientation, mental health training, and access to expert consultation as needed.

114. **D.** The Community Mental Health Centers Act of 1963 had a revolutionary impact by changing the direction of psychiatric nursing and expanding the role of the psychiatric nurse. Undergraduate courses in psychiatric nursing were first required in 1955.

115. **B.** The other two required services are partial hospitalization (day or night programs) and consultation and educational services to community agencies, groups, and individuals.

116. **D.** Thus, in some remote rural areas, the geographical boundaries containing a minimum population may be measured in hundreds of square miles, while in densely populated urban areas, a maximum population may exist in less than 100 square blocks.

117. **D.** The term catchment area is borrowed from the phrase used to describe reservoirs which catch water runoff after storms.

118. **D.** The WHO committee recommended (1) local emergency services with skilled medical and nursing staff (2) adequate and prompt psychiatric services with easy access to care where there is no other medical emergency service and follow-up psychiatric care. Members of the same psychiatric team should work in both emergency and follow-up care.

119. **B.** The Joint Commission on Mental Health of Children studied young people up to twenty-five years of age. The boundary was extended as far as twenty-five because society today often demands of adolescents long periods of educational and vocational preparation prior to their assuming adult responsibilities.

120. **D.** Only 7% of children needing treatment in the U.S. receive care. The Joint Commission sees this as clear indication for planning preventive strategies around developmental tasks and advocates treatment and preventive programs.

121. **C.** Orthopsychiatry places emphasis on preventive techniques to promote healthy emotional growth and development, particularly of children.

122. **C.** The I.C.D. is subscribed to by all WHO member nations who may assign their own terms to each I.C.D. category.

123. **B.** In 1966, the Center for Studies of Schizophrenia was organized in the National Institute of Mental Health. Its major goal is to coordinate the efforts of research, training, and service throughout the U.S.

124. **A.** The U.S. Department of Justice provided funds for two detoxification centers in demonstrative projects. They are located in St. Louis and Washington, D.C. These are to replace the punitive approach to alcoholism.

125. **B.** Founded in 1967, the American Association of Suicidology is the first nationwide organization. It stimulates research, education, and training in suicidology.

126. **D.** During the nineteenth century, one of the hospitals attached to the Fliedners group in Kaiserswerth was for the mentally ill; it probably was the first hospital for mentally ill patients in which trained nurses worked.

127. **A.** Descriptive diagnoses are usually taken from the American Psychiatric Association's *D.S.M. II.*

128. **B.** Linda Richards was America's first professional psychiatric nurse as well as the first American graduate nurse.

129. **D.** *Nursing Mental Diseases* by Harriet Bailey was published by Macmillan Company in 1920.

130. **C.** Under the vision and leadership of Dr. Esther Garrison, significant and remarkable accomplishments were made in psychiatric nursing. The 1946 National Mental Health Act provided the funds for which Dr. Garrison gave the direction for the field of psychiatric nursing.

131. **B.** Linda Richards was the first American graduate psychiatric nurse. Dorothea Lynde Dix, a school teacher, played a major role in mental health reform.

132. **D.** Psychoanalytic patients were usually treated in the analyst's office as private patients. However, when psychoanalytic theory became generally accepted and part of the curriculum in medical schools, psychiatric nurses practicing in units of teaching hospitals became aware of the value of this body of knowledge for psychiatric nursing education and practice.

133. **A.** Psychiatric nursing is indebted to Gwen Tudor for the first use of relationship theory as a technique applicable to the nursing care of psy-

chiatric patients. Her paper "A Sociopsychiatric Nursing Intervention in a Problem of Mutual Withdrawal on a Mental Hospital Ward" published in 1952, describes her use of this form of therapy.

134. **C.** Mellow's theoretical framework of nursing therapy draws on psychoanalytic theory in the sense that an intensive, symbiotic relationship is developed between the nurse and patient.

135. **B.** Hildegard Peplau in an article "Interpersonal Techniques: The Crux of Psychiatric Nursing," and Claire M. Fagin in "Psychotherapeutic Nursing" attempted to define the role of the psychiatric nurse.

136. **D.** Peplau considers as psychiatric nurses those who are specialists with advanced education. She bases this on the assumption that the difficulties in living which lead up to mental illness are subject to investigation and control by the patient with professional counseling assistance. Formal knowledge of counseling procedure is essential for the more general type of approach which is useful in very brief relationships with patients.

137. **D.** A clinical specialist in psychiatric nursing is prepared to perform the roles in all four areas.

138. **B.** Clinical specialization in psychiatric nursing is based on master's degree preparation in this clinical area.

139. **E.** Render published a textbook for psychiatric nurses which was one of the first to emphasize the nurse-patient relationship and contained no psychiatry except that related to nursing.

140. **D.** Dr. Peplau published the first systematic framework for psychiatric nursing.

141. **A.** Orlando's systematic theoretical approach, following 10 years after Peplau's publication, stimulated a flurry of publications based on Orlando's system.

142. **C.** Ujhely's book is a sociocultural analysis of the nurse-patient relationship.

143. **B.** Marram's book, published in 1973, was one of the first nursing texts to deal in depth with group concepts.

CHAPTER II

Developmental Status and Nursing Intervention

INTRODUCTION

Psychological development is an orderly process in human development. Tasks and tools, as well as developmental stages, can be identified throughout the life cycle. Normal growth and development, developmental crisis, psychological defense mechanisms, and the mental and developmental status examination will be reviewed in this chapter. Several developmental models will be presented with their concomitant psychobiological and sociocultural principles. The concept of anxiety and defenses against anxiety are areas that will be stressed as they play an integral role in psychiatric disorders. Nurses need to know and understand normal processes of the human psyche in order to recognize strengths, potential problems, and actual problems. Thus, the process and content of assessing mental and developmental status will be emphasized. It is this assessment that provides information for the data base from which nurses plan their interventions.

A. Normal Growth and Development and Developmental Crises

Directions: For each of the following multiple choice questions, select the ONE most appropriate answer.

1. Which of the following described a hierarchy of developmental stages that utilizes Freud's psychosexual themes?

   A. Anna Freud
   B. Robert Havighurst
   C. Erik Erikson
   D. Erich Fromm   (13:12–13)

2. Development characterized by an orderly sequence at particular stages, each depending upon the other for successful completion is called

   A. orthogenesis
   B. individuating maturation
   C. sensory motor development
   D. epigenesis   (1:4)

3. All of the following statements about Erikson's Eight Stages of Psychosocial Development are accurate *except*

   A. it takes into account the role of the society as well as the individual
   B. it is an example of how the intricacies of biological organization are matched by social organization
   C. the polarities, as in trust vs. mistrust, are either/or situations
   D. it theorizes that failures at one stage of development can be rectified by successes at later stages   (33:78–9)

4. According to Maslow, man's needs considered basic to growth and development emerge in what order?

    a. safety needs
    b. love needs
    c. physiological drives
    d. self-actualization needs
    e. esteem needs

    A. a, b, c, d, and e
    B. a, c, b, d, and e
    C. c, a, b, d, and e
    D. c, a, b, e, and d   (29:142–44)

5. Which of the following personal characteristics are influenced by genetic factors?

    a. numerical and verbal fluency
    b. hand dexterity
    c. social inversion
    d. activity and vigor

    A. a and b
    B. b and d
    C. a, b, and d
    D. a, b, c, and d   (18:66)

6. Which of the following statements regarding developmental tasks and levels is/are true?

    A. The task accomplished in each developmental stage must be reinforced or reaffirmed throughout the person's life
    B. If a developmental stage is left before partial completion, the person is handicapped in his later adjustments to life
    C. Although developmental tasks occur in a similar pattern, the chronological age of a person can't be equated with his developmental age
    D. all of the above   (29:153)

7. All of the following statements regarding Erikson's psychosocial theory of development are true *except*

    A. it builds solidly on Freudian analytic theory and is an extension of it
    B. it emphasizes the crucial role of the ego through the life cycle

    C. it is primarily concerned with the concept of "identity"
    D. it is a less optimistic theory than Freud's because of its focus on developmental tasks   (33:77–8)

8. Events that may influence psychosexual maturation include

    a. maternal absence
    b. birth of siblings
    c. deaths in the immediate family
    d. individual traumatic experiences

    A. a and b
    B. a, c, and d
    C. b, c, and d
    D. a, b, c, and d   (13:9)

9. The concept of critical periods of development refer to

    A. specific periods of the life cycle
    B. infancy through adolescence
    C. developmental time limits
    D. universal crises such as birth and death   (18:67)

Directions: MATCH the following numbered items (skills) with the most appropriate lettered items (developmental period).

Questions 10 to 19

10. Vocabulary increase is greatest   (14:33)
11. Peekaboo phenomenon   (14:53)
12. Socialized speech begins   (14:34)
13. Learns to perceive right from wrong   (14:34)
14. Hypothetical reasoning is possible   (14:34)
15. Language is egocentric   (14:33)
16. Intuitive stage   (14:34)
17. Learns relationships to external object   (14:33)
18. Knows that pouring water from short glass to tall glass does not change amount of water   (14:34)
19. Thinks logically   (14:34)

    A. Birth to 2 years
    B. 2 to 7 years
    C. 7 to 11 years
    D. 11 to 15 years

Directions: For each of the following multiple choice questions, select the ONE most appropriate answer.

20. The major portion of intellectual development takes place from

    A. conception to four years
    B. four to eight years
    C. eight to twelve years
    D. twelve to twenty-one years   (26:509)

21. Symbiosis is to independence as

    A. isolation is to loneliness
    B. isophilic is to heterophilic
    C. self respect is to identity
    D. mutuality is to collaboration   (10:417)

22. Competition, compromise, and cooperation are tools that become available to the person at the age of

    A. 2 to 6 years
    B. 6 to 9 years
    C. 9 to 12 years
    D. 12 to 18 years   (14:22)

23. Capacity to love, consensual validation, and collaboration are tools that become available at

    A. 6 to 9 years
    B. 9 to 12 years
    C. 12 to 15 years
    D. 15 to 18 years   (14:24)

24. Collaboration means the

    A. altering of one's behavior to meet the goals of another
    B. identification of another's behavior so that he can alter it to meet one's own goals
    C. mutual altering of behavior by two people to meet shared goals
    D. identification of similar behavior by two people to meet separate goals
                                         (29:98)

25. The subjectively experienced emotion which is characterized by feelings of vague, unexplained discomfort and apprehension is called

    A. stress
    B. anxiety
    C. fear
    D. panic   (29:158–59)

26. Mild anxiety is characterized by all of the following *except*

    A. a greater awareness of external stimuli
    B. a decrease in perceptual field
    C. a feeling of restlessness
    D. an increased ability to learn   (29:160)

27. Which of the following symptoms differentiates severe anxiety from moderate anxiety?

    A. a decrease in the perceptual field
    B. a tendency to concentrate on specific details rather than the whole
    C. a decrease in the ability to learn
    D. a feeling of dread or horror   (29:160)

28. Mr. and Mrs. Jensen lost their home in a flood. They are presently residing in a church with other victims of the disaster. Mrs. Jensen is frequently observed sitting alone and unresponsive to her surroundings. When she attempts to converse, she begins to cry. One would expect that Mrs. Jensen will

    A. resume her usual emotional responses when she is relocated
    B. progress into a depression as her home is lost forever
    C. adjust according to her adaptive capacity before the catastrophe
    D. develop overwhelming fears of floods
                                         (26:487)

29. Which of the following responses is the most appropriate for the nurse who is working with a person in a state of panic?

    A. "Can you tell me a little bit about what it is that is frightening you, Mr. Jacobs?"

B. "You look as if you are frozen to that spot. What are you feeling, Mr. Jacobs?"

C. "Let's take a walk down to the Occupational Therapy Room, Mr. Jacobs."

D. "Sit down. I will stay with you."

(29:160–61)

30. Alterations in the level of consciousness and/or in awareness of self may be precipated by

    a. direct injury to the brain
    b. hypoglycemia
    c. narcotics or alcohol
    d. loss of body part
    e. emotional stress

A. a and b
B. c
C. a, b, and c
D. a, b, c, d, and e (29:169)

31. Conflicts may be

    a. fully conscious
    b. partly conscious
    c. partly unconscious
    d. completely unconscious

A. b and c
B. b, c, and d
C. a and d
D. a, b, c, and d (21:79)

32. Sensory deprivation is apt to produce hallucinations that are

A. tactile
B. olfactory
C. visual
D. auditory (13:300)

33. Components of alienation include

    a. powerlessness
    b. normlessness
    c. meaninglessness
    d. social isolation

A. a and d
B. c and d

C. a and c
D. a, b, c, and d (13:175)

34. Studies of American class structure have suggested

A. the division of labor is more specialized in the lower-class family than in the middle-class family
B. the division of labor is most highly specialized in the middle-class family
C. child rearing is most apt to be shared by parents in an upper-class family
D. child rearing is most apt to be shared by parents in a lower-class family (29:152)

35. The first perceptions of the infant are

A. tactile
B. auditory
C. visual
D. olfactory (13:183)

36. Social smiling in the infant begins at about

A. birth to 2 weeks
B. 2 to 8 weeks
C. 12 to 24 weeks
D. 24 to 36 weeks (24:311)

37. Eighth month anxiety is a social landmark related to

A. attachment behavior
B. regressive behavior
C. the mother's warmth
D. depressive behavior (33:169)

38. A ten-month-old infant would not be expected to be able to

A. make babbling sounds
B. sit independently
C. show fear of strangers
D. say mama appropriately (24:307)

39. The infant begins to find a new face unpleasant at the age of

A. one to six months
B. eight to twelve months
C. six to eight months
D. twelve to eighteen months (18:69)

40. The nursery nurse who demonstrates the bathing and feeding of infants to new mothers is utilizing strategies of

    A. primary prevention
    B. secondary prevention
    C. corrective intervention
    D. reinforcement   (18:61)

41. Harlow's studies indicate that the attachment process is

    A. strictly a learned response on the part of the infant
    B. a learned response on the part of both mother and infant
    C. dependent entirely on the mother's ability to interpret the infant's cues
    D. affected by the infant's inborn capacity to emit attachment behavior   (18:68)

42. Which of the following are examples of attachment behavior of the infant?

    a. clinging
    b. smiling
    c. vocalization
    d. scanning

    A. a and c
    B. b and d
    C. a, c, and d
    D. a, b, c, and d   (18:68)

43. Which of the following behavior on the part of a mother of a premature infant indicates a higher probability of family crisis?

    A. awareness of the danger of losing the infant
    B. acknowledged failure in her ability to deliver a mature infant
    C. lack of questioning behavior about the infant's well-being
    D. interest in the infant's special needs   (1:68)

44. Possible emotional causes of abnormal crying despite the mother's presence include

    a. chronic ignoring of crying by the mother

    b. oversolicitous behavior by the mother
    c. overtense, jerky, physical handling
    d. hunger, cold, wet diaper

    A. a and c
    B. a, c, and d
    C. a, b, and c
    D. b, c, and d   (21:362)

45. An infant fed with a propped bottle and a large nipple hole might be expected to develop

    A. a severe personality disorder
    B. feelings of frustration
    C. traits of stinginess and compulsiveness
    D. a psychotic disorder   (21:99)

46. Transient disturbances in infancy include psychogenically based symptoms such as

    a. undue apathy
    b. disturbances of sleeping
    c. eating problems
    d. phobias

    A. a
    B. b and c
    C. a, b, and c
    D. b, c, and d   (20:538)

47. Examples of oral character traits are

    A. dependency and egocentricity
    B. miserliness and gullibility
    C. conformity and philanthropy
    D. sarcasm and creativity   (20:50)

48. The nurse would suspect the presence of a physiological or psychological problem if the child fails to utilize speech by

    A. 18 months
    B. 24 months
    C. 36 months
    D. 42 months   (20:62)

49. Which of the following statements about autistic invention are true?

a. it is the use of highly personal meanings for words and events
b. it is normally used by children
c. it is never used by normal persons
d. it is frequently used by schizophrenic patients

A. a and b
B. a, c, and d
C. a and d
D. a, b, and d   (9:11–12)

50. In a study of child abuse, mothers who abuse their children were found to feel that a child should know right from wrong by

A. 6 months
B. 12 months
C. 18 months
D. 24 months   (10:382)

51. Abusive mothers tend to be

A. lower class
B. socially active
C. isolated
D. members of civic groups   (10:382)

52. In cases of child abuse, there is a relationship between social class and

A. the incidence of abuse
B. the reason for discipline
C. age for discipline
D. the manner of discipline   (10:382)

53. In caring for a child that the nurse suspects has been the victim of parental abuse, the nurse should

a. speak softly to the child and maintain slight physical contact
b. tell the child that he is safe
c. question the parents with the child present
d. inform the parents that a report will have to be made

A. a and b
B. a and c
C. b and d
D. a, b, and d   (31:136–37)

54. Bowlby demonstrated patterns of reaction in two-year-old children who were hospitalized. The behavior observed included

A. crying, searching, and cooperating
B. apathy
C. withdrawal
D. all of the above   (21:363–64)

55. According to Bowlby's research with hospitalized two-year-olds, the child can recover without serious residual effects if an adequate mother substitute takes over before the conclusion of

A. the protest phase
B. the despair phase
C. the detachment phase
D. all of the above   (21:364)

56. When the physical exam and urinalysis are normal, what percentage of cases of enuresis in children over 4 years of age is due to emotional tension?

A. 25%
B. 50%
C. 75%
D. 99%   (2:370)

57. Miss Cook, a staff nurse, finds Paul and Mary ages 3 and 4, in the bathroom examining each other's anatomy and comparing the differences. The children seem unconcerned that Miss Cook found them. Which behavior on Miss Cook's part indicates an understanding of this developmental stage?

A. to tell the children that boys and girls are not allowed to be in the bathroom together
B. to tell the children that little boys and little girls should not look at one another
C. to tell the children to get dressed and return to activities
D. to pretend that she did not notice the behavior   (33:137)

58. Paul, age 3, is brought to well-child clinic by his mother. Mrs. Ivring complains that Paul has begun to suck his thumb constantly and wet his bed since the arrival of his baby sister. His behavior is best described as

    A.   repressed
    B.   retarded
    C.   regressed
    D.   fixated   (21:505)

59. At this time, Paul can best be helped if his mother

    A.   gives him a bottle when she gives the baby one
    B.   explains that he's no longer a baby
    C.   get him up to urinate during the night
    D.   gives him special attention   (2:338)

60. Johnny, age four, has been experiencing nightmares for several months. His mother reports to the nurse that Johnny is comforted by allowing him into bed with her while her husband takes Johnny's bed. The nurse should assess

    A.   the developmental significance of this behavior
    B.   the knowledge level of the mother
    C.   the frequency of the nightmares
    D.   all of the above   (21:371)

61. The nurse has assessed that Johnny's behavior is within normal limits, that is, that his anxiety is not excessive. She decides to suggest an alternative solution to that proposed by the parents. The nurse recognizes that the parents' behavior is likely to

    A.   intensify an unconscious conflict on Johnny's part
    B.   cause manipulation on Johnny's part
    C.   predispose Johnny to homosexual behavior
    D.   intensify feelings of sibling rivalry
                                              (21:371)

62. The nurse might suggest to Johnny's mother that Johnny may need to

    a.   refrain from eating before bedtime
    b.   talk out his fears with his parents

    c.   go back to sleep in his own bed
    d.   sleep with his father rather than his mother

    A.   a, b, and c
    B.   b and d
    C.   a and d
    D.   b and c   (21:371)

63. Which of the following would Erikson regard as typical for 4-1/2-year-old Johnny?

    A.   constant chattering
    B.   concern with bowel movements
    C.   wish to be cuddled
    D.   tendency to shyness   (33:80–1)

64. A five-year-old child's curiosity about his sexual organs is a sign of

    A.   abnormal development
    B.   normal development
    C.   pathogical sexual drives
    D.   faulty sexual identity   (24:408)

65. Bryon becomes nauseated every school morning but on Saturdays and Sundays manifests no symptoms. Bryon probably has a/an

    A.   propensity toward delinquency
    B.   authoritarian teacher
    C.   school phobia
    D.   severe mental disorder   (6:II:121)

66. Which of the following statements about children with school phobia are true?

    a.   these children are usually of average intelligence
    b.   the parents of these children are achievement-oriented
    c.   their parents are indifferent to school
    d.   these children respect authority

    A.   a and d
    B.   b and d
    C.   a and c
    D.   a, b, and d   (13:15)

67. In working with the child under ten with school phobia, the most appropriate nursing intervention is to

    A. ignore the absence from school and talk with the mother
    B. encourage the mother to accompany the child to school
    C. help the child return to school as soon as possible
    D. encourage the school to change the child's teacher   (13:15)

68. The underlying psychopathology of school phobia is related to

    A. unresolved oedipal strivings
    B. separation
    C. overly rigid toilet training
    D. minimal brain dysfunction   (4:88)

69. In children over the age of ten who experience school phobias, the nurse should

    A. enforce school attendance
    B. initiate a psychiatric referral
    C. accompany the child to school
    D. suspect depressive behavior   (2:165)

70. Which of the following behaviors seen in the juvenile era is an example of social accommodation?

    A. developing satisfactory play habits
    B. seeing his parents as less godlike
    C. winning his teacher's recognition
    D. moving from inductive to deductive reasoning   (14:29)

71. Excessive rebelliousness on the part of a child in latency is typically the result of

    a. overpermissive parenting
    b. overcontrolling parenting
    c. peer pressure
    d. sibling rivalry

    A. a and c
    B. a and b
    C. b and c
    D. b and d   (21:369)

72. Examples of habit disturbances of childhood include all of the following *except*

    A. nail-biting
    B. enuresis
    C. masturbation
    D. stealing   (26:488)

73. Which of the following neuroses is commonly seen in children under five years of age?

    A. reactive depression
    B. conversion reaction
    C. phobias
    D. anxiety reaction   (6:120–22)

74. Which of the following on the part of adolescents can be seen as normal developmental affects and behaviors?

    a. short periods of messiness and obstinacy
    b. arrogance and grandiosity
    c. destruction of property
    d. frank rebellion

    A. a and d
    B. b and d
    C. a and b
    D. b and c   (6:II:226–28)

75. According to Erikson, the components of a sense of identity are

    a. a feeling of being at home in one's body
    b. a sense of "knowing where one is going"
    c. an inner certainty of anticipated recognition from those who count
    d. a readiness to face the challenges of the adult world

    A. a
    B. a and c
    C. b and d
    D. a, b, c, and d   (33:80)

76. By the end of adolescence, which of the following characterize the normal adolescent?

    A. an established sexual identity
    B. acquisition of independence
    C. a personal moral value system
    D. all of the above   (33:80–1, 229)

77. The term, self-diffusion, as used by Erikson means

    A. isolation
    B. overidentification
    C. self-absorption
    D. autonomy   (29:156–57)

78. Which of the following statements about adolescent turmoil is generally agreed to as accurate?

    A. adolescent turmoil is a frequent phenomenon
    B. adolescent turmoil is a normal developmental process
    C. adolescent turmoil is an infrequent phenomenon
    D. adolescent turmoil reflects psychopathology   (18:105)

79. According to Erikson, the central conflict of the young adult is

    A. identity vs. role diffusion
    B. generativity vs. stagnation
    C. intimacy vs. isolation
    D. initiative vs. guilt   (33:80–1)

80. Which of the following is *not* a characteristic of early adulthood?

    A. peak physical and mental efficiency
    B. major adjustment to new life patterns
    C. decreasing concern with vocation
    D. developing new interests and attitudes   (33:80–1)

81. Which of the following are sexual myths or common misconceptions?

    a. nocturnal emissions (wet dreams) are indicators of sexual disorders
    b. a mature sexual relationship requires the male and female to achieve simultaneous orgasm
    c. it is dangerous to have intercourse during menstruation
    d. it is "unnatural" for a woman to have as strong a desire for sex as a man

    A. a
    B. c
    C. b and d
    D. a, b, c, and d   (33:132–33)

82. The cyclic changes in mood associated with menstruation indicate

    A. an inability to accept oneself as a woman
    B. a poor relationship with one's mother
    C. a normal response to hormonal alterations
    D. frustrated maternal needs   (21:122)

83. According to Havighurst, paying taxes, voting, and involvement in community affairs are tasks initiated in

    A. adolescence
    B. early adulthood
    C. middle age
    D. later maturity   (13:18–21)

Questions 84 to 85

Miss Bush, a 25-year-old secretary, asks your advice about her conflicting emotions regarding marriage.

84. Miss Bush appears to be grappling with

    A. an identity crisis
    B. an intimacy-isolation crisis
    C. feelings of inferiority
    D. a depressive episode   (33:80–1)

85. In talking with Miss Bush, she dwells on the present and has few plans made for the future. This is an example of

A. immaturity
B. flight from reality
C. age appropriate behavior
D. avoidance   (7:163)

86. In Western society, divorce has become an increasingly common occurrence. The largest proportion of divorces occurs

    a. in the early years of marriage
    b. in the middle years of marriage
    c. among childless couples
    d. among couples who have children

A. a and c
B. a and d
C. b and c
D. b and d   (1:93)

87. Divorces are more common among couples who

A. come from an urban background
B. come from a rural background
C. had a long engagement
D. have the same religious beliefs   (1:93)

88. In instances where *both* parties have been divorced two or more times, the ratio of remarriage

A. is lower than the normal rate
B. falls within the normal rate
C. is higher than the normal rate
D. is twice as high as the normal rate (1:94)

89. The peak of divorces occurs in the

A. first year of marriage
B. second year of marriage
C. eighteenth year of marriage
D. twenty-second year of marriage   (1:93)

Directions: Match the following numbered items with letter of the most appropriate phase of mourning.

Questions 90 to 97

90. Anger at the doctor   (27:II:4–8)
91. Open casket   (27:II:4–8)
92. Phase of promiscuity   (27:II:4–8)
93. "Oh no, I don't believe it"   (27:II:4–8)

94. Confusion and indifference   (27:II:4–8)
95. Sobbing   (27:II:4–8)
96. Remarriage   (27:II:4–8)
97. Belief in reunion in heaven   (27:II:4–8)

A. Denial
B. Rageful protest
C. Cry for help
D. Despair
E. Detachment and recovery

Directions: For each of the following multiple choice questions, select the ONE most appropriate answer.

98. In the healthy person, the involutional period of life marks the loss of

A. sexual drives
B. reproductive abilities
C. a spouse
D. sexual attractiveness   (2:124)

99. Which of the following is an adjustment reaction of old age?

A. senescence
B. low morale following retirement
C. involutional depression
D. early morning awakening   (26:488)

100. According to Erikson, the central task of senescence is that of

A. intimacy vs. isolation
B. independence vs. dependence
C. generativity vs. stagnation
D. ego integrity vs. despair   (33:80–1)

101. The desire for intergenerational contact is

A. both greatly desired and expected by older people
B. possibly less extensive and intensive on the part of the aged than is generally believed
C. more desired by the old due to their increased dependence upon the younger generation
D. increased and sustained among the aged through social welfare and social security   (8:10–11)

102. The statement that, "as the individual ages, his life space tends to constrict and he experiences a general curtailment of involvement in social life," is an example of which of the following theories of aging?

   A. aging as a subculture
   B. aging as a part of the life course
   C. aging as disengagement
   D. aging as regression   (8:18)

103. The concept of generativity as described by Erikson is illustrated by

   A. the concern of a parent for the child's livelihood
   B. the concern of a teacher for the student's learning
   C. the concern of a nurse for the client's health
   D. all of the above   (33:80–1)

104. The life review, a phenomenon of old age, is

   A. due to the loss of recent memory
   B. one of the cardinal signs of senility
   C. is seen only in the elderly
   D. a universal mental process   (13:25)

105. The failure to achieve the task of generativity results in a state of

   A. stagnation
   B. pseudo-intimacy
   C. regression
   D. psychological invalidism   (33:80–1)

106. Studies on aging have indicated that

   A. psychological aging and physical aging are always parallel
   B. aging increases the susceptibility to illness
   C. the elderly use more physician services but have fewer hospital admissions than younger age groups
   D. all of the above   (8:54)

107. Recent studies have shown that the elderly who have a history of extensive social contact with their peers tend to

   A. be easily influenced by their peers in the evaluation of their own health
   B. be more objective in evaluating their own health status
   C. be less objective in evaluating their own health status
   D. avoid peers who are ill   (8:86)

108. Senescence can be distinguished from earlier stages in human development in that

   A. senescence brings about dramatic changes in personality
   B. senescence is the only stage of life in which no growth occurs
   C. senescence is a movement toward a final end
   D. senescence is primarily a period of living in the past   (8:125)

109. Which of the following statements about aging is true?

   A. the majority of the aged population live in some type of institution
   B. old age is a kind of second childhood
   C. most older people prefer to live apart from their own children but close enough to see them often
   D. aged persons have no sex life   (8:63–6)

110. Reasons why the elderly frequently complain about the food served to them include

   a. a marked decrease in the number of taste buds
   b. an increased ability to smell
   c. a loss of permanent teeth and deterioration of gums
   d. an increase in the saliva secretion which increases intestinal motility

   A. a only
   B. a and c
   C. b and c
   D. all of the above   (8:60–1)

111. Which of the following statements is/are true regarding hearing and the aged?

a. hearing becomes less acute with age
b. there is an increase in hearing for high frequencies and a decrease for low frequencies
c. women tend to have a greater hearing loss than men
d. hearing aids are less easily accepted than eye glasses

A. a only
B. a and b
C. b and c
D. a and d   (8:112–13)

112. The learning capacity of the aged is

A. decreased because of inability to learn new knowledge
B. unaffected by age
C. increased when anxiety is high and motivation is high
D. much the same as for younger people in terms of content capable of being learned   (8:117–18)

113. The disengagement process in aging is characterized by an increased

A. closeness between the individual and his social system
B. dissatisfaction with one's life
C. ability to view one's own death objectively
D. dependence on other people for emotional support   (8:18)

B. Psychological Defense Mechanisms

Directions: For each of the following multiple choice questions, select the ONE most appropriate answer.

114. The principle that every act of human behavior has its cause, or source, in the history and experience of the individual is called

A. symbolic identification
B. genetic determinism
C. psychic determinism
D. projective identification   (1:2–3)

115. The key differentiating factors between "coping" and adaptation are

A. ego defenses vs. environmental resources
B. independence vs. dependence
C. "buying time" vs. long term adjustment
D. psychological change vs. physiological change   (32:478)

116. Anxiety serves to

A. provide a "warning signal"
B. alert the human organism of an impending threat
C. provide stimulation for normal pursuits
D. all of the above   (29:158–60)

117. Conflict is caused by

A. ambivalence
B. trauma
C. stress
D. all of the above   (16:19)

118. Which of the following factors influence the aim and the object of a basic drive?

a. unconscious cultural factors
b. conscious cultural factors
c. unconscious psychological factors
d. conscious psychological factors

A. a and c
B. b and d
C. b, c, and d
D. a, b, c, and d   (21:64)

119. Ego functioning is influenced by the

a. id
b. superego
c. social environment
d. reality principle

A. a and b
B. a, b, and c
C. a, b, and d
D. a, b, c, and d   (20:43–5)

120. Which of the following statements about fixation is *not* accurate?

    A. fixation results in a more favorable prognosis than regression
    B. it is difficult to distinguish between regressed behavior and fixated behavior
    C. fixation can result from excessive gratification of needs
    D. fixation can result from excessive frustration of needs   (21:106)

121. If a person is comfortable with his presenting symptoms, they are called

    A. ego alien
    B. ego syntonic
    C. ego dystonic
    D. none of the above   (32:247–50)

122. Ambivalent feelings contribute to emotional illness when they are

    a. strong
    b. unconscious
    c. conscious
    d. toward significant others

    A. a and d
    B. a and b
    C. b and d
    D. a, b, c, and d   (2:62)

123. The ego solves the problems of controlling id impulses by

    A. the use of a variety of mental mechanisms
    B. repression of all unacceptable impulses
    C. sublimation of all unacceptable impulses
    D. the use of reaction formation   (18:232)

124. A person who becomes tense when frustrated is

    A. an extravert
    B. neurotic
    C. normal
    D. an introvert   (26:138)

125. Typically, fixation involves the development of the

    a. intellectual functions
    b. sexual drives
    c. social drives
    d. motor skills

    A. a and d
    B. a and b
    C. b and c
    D. c and d   (21:98–100)

126. Illusions can be caused by

    a. anxiety
    b. fatigue
    c. intoxication
    d. isolation

    A. a and d
    B. b and c
    C. a, c, and d
    D. a, b, c, and d   (10:235)

127. Ego defense mechanisms serve to

    a. minimize anxiety
    b. protect the ego
    c. manage aggressive impulses
    d. increase anxiety

    A. a, b, and c
    B. a and b
    C. b and c
    D. a, b, c, and d   (20:68)

128. The unconscious process by which parental attitudes are taken into one's self concept is called

    A. sublimation
    B. rationalization
    C. introjection
    D. fixation   (26:148)

129. Jane is furious at her head nurse for always assigning her to the "most difficult" patients. She says nothing to the head nurse but when arriving home for dinner, Jane has a big argument with her roommate about whose turn it was to shop for dinner. Jane is

A. projecting
B. identifying
C. rationalizing
D. displacing   (10:411)

130. Projection, as a defense mechanism, is not utilized by

A. neurotic patients
B. alcoholic patients
C. depressed patients
D. drug addicts   (10:187)

131. Mrs. Rogers has an obsessive need to nag her son about his school work. She justifies her behavior by saying that there is no other way that her son will get through high school. Mrs. Rogers is

A. projecting
B. compensating
C. rationalizing
D. identifying   (10:416)

132. On the night Nancy plans to complete her term paper for a course she finds particularly difficult, she develops a severe cramp in her right hand. Nancy is using the defense mechanism of

A. displacement
B. conversion
C. suppression
D. dissociation   (10:410)

133. Hero worship is an example of

A. incorporation
B. introjection
C. identification
D. empathy   (20:72–4)

134. An explanation which contains an element of truth but which is so unduly emphasized so as to conceal the essential prompting motive is known as the defense mechanism of

A. suppression
B. denial
C. symbolization
D. rationalization   (20:75–6)

135. Hypocrisy is the conscious counterpart of which of the following unconscious defense mechanisms?

A. sublimation
B. denial
C. reaction formation
D. projection   (20:74)

136. An elderly patient plans to return home after a stroke without considering that paralysis makes it impossible to climb the stairs to the apartment. This is an example of

A. rationalization
B. suppression
C. denial
D. idealization   (20:83)

137. A nurse intensely dislikes an aide. Without being aware of doing so, the nurse goes out of her way not to be critical and gives him special privileges. This is an example of

A. undoing
B. displacement
C. suppression
D. reaction formation   (4:83)

138. A nurse is angered by a patient and suppresses her anger. She goes home and argues with her husband about an incident she usually would have ignored. This is an example of the defense mechanism of

A. repression
B. reaction formation
C. displacement
D. aim inhibition   (20:77)

139. A young man is thinking about a date he has planned and finds he cannot concentrate on his studies. He decides to put the date out of his mind until after he has studied. This is an example of

A. repression
B. denial
C. suppression
D. sublimation   (20:71)

Directions: Each group of numbered words or phrases is followed by a list of lettered statements. MATCH the lettered statement most closely associated with the numbered word or phrase.

Questions 140 to 149

140. A man with strong sexual drives writes poetry (26:149)
141. A boy who wishes to hit his father and develops paralysis of the arm (26:150)
142. A boy who feels hostile towards his sister is very polite to her (26:147)
143. A man is angry with his wife and spanks his daughter (26:148)
144. A patient says to the nurse "You're an iceberg" (26:151)
145. The patient says, "I am Napoleon" (26:150)
146. "I'd rather not talk about it" (26:146)
147. A man with diabetes continues to eat whatever he likes (26:147)
148. A boy kicks his sister and says "I'm sorry" (26:151)
149. "I could have passed the test if I had tried" (26:146)

    A. Suppression
    B. Conversion
    C. Undoing
    D. Condensation
    E. Displacement
    F. Sublimation
    G. Denial
    H. Rationalization
    I. Reaction formation
    J. Symbolism

Directions: For each of the following multiple choice questions, select the ONE most appropriate answer.

150. Tommy hits his young brother and then quickly goes and gets his favorite toy to give to him. This is an example of

    A. reaction formation
    B. displacement
    C. undoing
    D. compensation (20:426)

151. The student who unconsciously models himself after his favorite teacher and begins dressing and talking like him is exhibiting the mechanism of

    A. introjection
    B. compensation
    C. idealization
    D. identification (4:47)

152. Mrs. Clark, a very righteous woman, loses her temper with the grocer and makes some "unlady-like" remarks. When she returns home, she spends five minutes brushing her teeth. This is an example of

    A. dissociation
    B. undoing
    C. condensation
    D. symbolism (4:100)

153. The defense mechanism that figures most prominently in the symptoms of delusions and hallucinations is

    A. reaction formation
    B. sublimation
    C. projection
    D. compensation (4:77)

154. When we say "It's on the tip of my tongue," reference is being made to thoughts that are

    A. conscious
    B. preconscious
    C. unconscious
    D. blocked (21:43)

155. A college student becomes furious at what he feels is unfair treatment by his professor. He deems it unwise to be openly aggressive to him and finds himself becoming tense. After class, he goes to the gym and punches a punching bag viciously. Gradually the angry tension subsides. This is an example of

    A. sublimation
    B. suppression
    C. regression
    D. denial (21:71)

156. According to psychoanalytic theory, "love at first sight" is most likely a form of

    A. transference phenomenon
    B. positive identification
    C. narcissism
    D. projection   (21:427)

157. A person who has exhibited sadistic behavior begins to exhibit masochistic behavior. This is an example of

    A. reaction formation
    B. sublimation
    C. reversal
    D. undoing   (21:505)

158. Reversal differs from reaction formation with respect to

    A. attitude change
    B. behavior change
    C. consciousness of motivation
    D. stress factors   (21:103–04)

159. Sheila, age four, is tired and irritable. Her mother insists that she take a nap. Sheila becomes angry at her mother but is not aware of this. She exclaims, "You don't like me." The defense mechanism described is

    A. introjection
    B. suppression
    C. projection
    D. denial   (21:504)

160. Johnny, five years of age, has been promised that he will be going to the movies. The outing is cancelled because the film is postponed. Johnny is told this but later in the day, insists that the family is going to the movies. He is utilizing the defense mechanism of

    A. blocking
    B. suppression
    C. denial
    D. displacement   (26:147)

161. Defense mechanisms can be seen as coping devices whereby the person

    a. moves against others or a situation
    b. moves away from others or a situation
    c. moves forward and attempts to conform
    d. remains static

    A. a and b
    B. c and d
    C. a and d
    D. a, b, and c   (26:142–45)

162. Another label for reaction formation is

    A. compensation
    B. overcompensation
    C. substitution
    D. incorporation   (26:147)

163. The ego does not play a role in which of the following defense mechanisms?

    A. repression
    B. regression
    C. sublimation
    D. suppression   (21:106)

164. Observations of prisoners in German Concentration Camps who eventually copied the values and behavior of the Gestapo best illustrate the ego defense mechanism of

    A. projection
    B. introjection
    C. rationalization
    D. identification   (20:72)

165. Which of the following behaviors can be seen as defenses against loneliness?

    A. excessive planning
    B. increased productivity
    C. focusing
    D. self-appraisal   (27:II:58)

166. The client who experiences loneliness may attempt to establish contact with the nurse through

    A. hero worship
    B. role reversal
    C. somatic participation
    D. all of the above   (27:II:59–60)

167. The mechanism that is necessary for the process of identification is

    A. projection
    B. imitation
    C. introjection
    D. sublimation   (21:111)

168. Which of the following defenses accounts for ideas reaching the intensity of delusions?

    A. projection
    B. repression
    C. regression
    D. condensation   (21:278)

169. Which of the following is *not* considered an ego defense mechanism?

    A. sublimation
    B. undoing
    C. repression
    D. regression   (21:106)

170. Individuals exhibiting homosexual behavior usually show which of the following personality features?

    a. difficulty in reconciling dependent and assertive drives
    b. extreme feelings of failure
    c. an ambivalent maternal relationship
    d. a high frequency of being reared in a broken home

    A. a and b
    B. a, b, and c
    C. a, c, and d
    D. a, b, c, and d   (20:504)

C. Mental and Developmental Status Examinations

Directions: For each of the following multiple choice questions, select the ONE most appropriate answer.

Questions 171 to 181 refer to the two parts of this examination—the psychiatric history and the mental status exams.

Following Mrs. Peterson's admission to the hospital, the nurse did a psychiatric examination.

171. Although the psychiatric history (PH) and the mental status examination (MSE) are both part of a psychiatric examination, the PH differs from the MSE in that the PH

    A. focuses on the form of observable behavioral responses
    B. focuses on the content of individual experience
    C. emphasizes the here and now
    D. is the more objective of the two (32:529)

172. Mrs. Peterson interrupts the nurse in the middle of the history taking and says in a very loud voice, "One swallow doesn't make a summer." The most appropriate inference on the part of the nurse is that Mrs. Peterson

    A. is able to reason abstractly
    B. has been given a MSE before
    C. does not want her symptoms to be judged too harshly
    D. is probably psychotic   (32:92–3)

173. The purpose of the Mental Status Examination (MSE) is to provide an accurate description of the patient's current functioning. This record can be used

    A. as a base line for later comparisons
    B. as a standard for evaluating changes in past performance as inferred from history
    C. for comparisons between individuals in aiding psychodiagnosis
    D. all of the above   (32:529)

174. All of the following statements about the PH and the MSE are true *except*

    A. the cognitive testing of the MSE is usually done before the PH
    B. the PH is best collected in an open-ended fashion
    C. the MSE consists of more formalized questions than the PH
    D. data concerning the PH is sometimes ellicted when doing the MSE and vice-versa   (32:529–36)

175. Examples of data which might be recorded about kinetics include

     a. body build
     b. gait
     c. gestures
     d. physical defects

     A. a and b
     B. b and c
     C. c and d
     D. a and d   (32:529)

176. Mrs. Peterson tells the nurse that she is concerned her neighbors may be talking about her. This is an example of

     A. free-floating anxiety
     B. delusions of persecution
     C. depersonalization
     D. ideas of reference   (32:530–31)

177. The nurse tests for similarities by naming items that are the same or alike in certain ways and asks Mrs. Peterson in what way they are alike. This tests the patient's ability of

     A. abstract reasoning
     B. recent memory
     C. judgement
     D. orientation   (32:535)

178. Given twelve sets of similar items by the nurse, Mrs. Peterson correctly classifies seven of the similarities. The nurse would be correct if she concluded that Mrs. Peterson is intellectually

     A. below average
     B. average
     C. above average
     D. far above average   (32:535)

179. Tests of the cognitive functions are useful for

     A. obtaining a baseline for later comparisons
     B. distinguishing organic brain disease from the functional psychoses
     C. estimating intelligence
     D. all of the above   (32:532)

180. The nurse asks Mrs. Peterson to do serial 7's—that is, subtract 7's from 100 in serial fashion audibly and as fast as she can. This is a tool designed to test

     A. memory
     B. vocabulary
     C. judgement
     D. attention   (32:533)

181. Mrs. Peterson took 85 seconds to do this test and made five errors. The nurse should recognize that Mrs. Peterson's performance was

     A. excellent
     B. within normal limits
     C. marginal
     D. poor   (32:533)

182. When taking a psychiatric history, many parts of the mental status exam can be done simultaneously if the interviewer

     A. uses a standardized form or outline
     B. asks simple questions that can be answered "yes" or "no"
     C. follows a chronological order in gathering data
     D. allows the client to give a variety of spontaneous responses   (25:42)

183. The "process" of a psychiatric interview refers to

     A. the verbal communication of messages
     B. the nonverbal communication of messages
     C. the how and why of the participants' behavior
     D. the emotional reaction of the therapist   (25:8)

184. Examples of personality tests include the

     a. Rorschach test
     b. Thematic Apperception test
     c. Sentence Completion test
     d. Draw-A-Person test

     A. a and b
     B. c and d
     C. a, b, and d
     D. a, b, c, and d   (2:88–9)

185. In evaluating orientation in the client, the examiner needs to

    a. listen carefully to the client's remarks during the interview
    b. ask direct questions about orientation
    c. ask direct questions only if doubt exists about orientation after using indirect approaches
    d. avoid direct questions as these embarrass the client

    A. a and b
    B. a and c
    C. a and d
    D. b   (6:I:1176–77)

186. Which of the following questions is designed to focus on evaluating insight?

    A. Do you have any thoughts that you have difficulty getting rid of?
    B. Do you remember what 10 times 10 is?
    C. What do you think about most?
    D. What brought all this on?   (6:I:1175)

187. Which of the following factors affect the appropriateness of emotions?

    a. cultural differences in emotional expression
    b. feelings of shame regarding one's emotions
    c. the presence of a strong and lasting emotion
    d. misperceptions of other people

    A. a and b
    B. a, b, and c
    C. a and c
    D. a, b, c, and d   (6:I:1163)

188. The mental and emotional assessment can be *best* described as

    A. a criteria for assessing mental stability
    B. a picture of the emotional and mental functioning of the client
    C. the client's behavior in response to stress
    D. life events, attitudes, and adaptive responses   (32:529)

189. The area of "thought content" refers to

    A. the way the client thinks
    B. the quality of the client's fantasy life
    C. the ideas and fears constituting the substance of his thought
    D. the client's ability to plan his thinking toward the future   (20:158–59)

190. The client's mental state during the mental status assessment may be influenced by

    a. alterations of the client's emotional state induced by recent events
    b. the attitude of the client toward the interviewer
    c. the attitude of the client toward the interview
    d. the attitude of the interviewer toward the client

    A. a and d
    B. b and d
    C. a and c
    D. a, b, c, and d   (6:I:1160)

191. The best reason for ascertaining individual characteristics and assets when doing a psychiatric examination is because awareness of these areas

    A. encourages the client to feel at ease
    B. deemphasizes the clinical role of the interviewer
    C. influences the outcome of the illness
    D. is needed for one to do clinical research   (6:I:1158)

192. Psychiatric symptoms may be considered as

    a. exclusively defensive efforts
    b. disorders directly produced by a lesion or acquired during a stress
    c. efforts to compensate for disorders produced by a lesion or a stress
    d. efforts to counteract the lesion or stress

    A. a only
    B. b and d
    C. b, c, and d
    D. a, c, and d   (6:I:1158)

Directions: The Mental Status Exam is essential in making a diagnosis and dynamic formulation. MATCH the cognitive function being examined with the correct example of how you might test for it.

Questions 193 to 200

193. Orientation (32:532)
194. Attention and Concentration (32:532-33)
195. Memory (32:533)
196. Information (32:534)
197. Vocabulary (32:534)
198. Abstraction (32:534–35)
199. Judgement and Comprehension (32:535–36)
200. Perception and Coordination (32:536)

A. "Explain the proverb 'As the twig is bent, the tree's inclined.'"
B. Drop a pencil or magazine and observe if client notices
C. "What is today's date?"
D. "What did you have for lunch?"
E. "Why is it usually better to give money to an organized charity than to a street beggar?"
F. "What is a barometer?"
G. "Define or tell me the meaning of the following words: fable, apple, nuisance, plural, stanza, recede, seclude, and guillotine."
H. Have the patient copy a square, a diamond, and a row of dots on a piece of paper.

Directions: For each of the following multiple choice questions, select the ONE most appropriate answer.

201. In taking a psychiatric history, the interviewer obtains data which focuses upon the client's

A. maturational development and interpersonal reactions
B. affectivity and mood
C. general appearance
D. level of consciousness (20:152)

202. The psychiatric examination is useful in uncovering data under which of the following headings?

a. signs of major psychological disturbances

b. psychological factors which have a causative influence in a major physical illness
c. psychological reactions to the presence of another illness
d. psychological factors which interfere with the patient's cooperation in treatment

A. a and b
B. a and c
C. b, c, and d
D. a, b, c, and d (6:I:1157)

203. In gathering data for initial assessment, it is important for the nurse to be aware that the data will be

a. complete after several sessions
b. incomplete even after several sessions
c. the basis for tentative formulations about dynamics
d. complete if the interviewer is skilled and perceptive

A. a and c
B. b and c
C. c and d
D. a, c, and d (18:551)

204. In conducting an initial interview with an acutely psychotic client, it is most important that the nurse

A. gives messages of interest and support
B. be more structured in her format
C. be less structured in her format
D. demonstrate concern (18:548)

205. The interviewer notes that Miss Karns, a fashionably dressed 36-year-old woman, is attired neatly in a dress but is wearing stockings and sneakers. The interviewer should

A. refer vaguely to Miss Karns' interest in tennis
B. ask Miss Karns if she has had a recent orthopedic injury
C. note the incongruity between her attire and her footwear
D. regard this as unimportant and probably familial behavior (20:156)

Directions: Each group of numbered words or phrases is followed by a list of lettered statements. MATCH the lettered statement most closely associated with the numbered word or phrase in relation to ego functions.

Questions 206 to 210

206. "I fly off the handle frequently." (18:553)
207. "My brain is dead." (18:553)
208. "I wash my hands fifty times a day, I can't stop myself." (18:554)
209. "I know you can read my mind." (18:554)
210. "We think alike on everything and have for thirty years." (18:553)

    A. Relationship to Reality
    B. Regulation of Drives
    C. Object Relations
    D. Thought Process
    E. Defensive Functions

Directions: For each of the following multiple choice questions, select the ONE most appropriate answer.

211. Abnormalities of thought content include

    A. ambivalence
    B. delusions
    C. illusions
    D. hallucinations (6:I:1168)

212. What process does the following question attempt to identify? "Have you ever felt as if you were not yourself, or as if you had changed so that you couldn't recognize yourself?"

    A. delusions
    B. depersonalization
    C. nihilistic thinking
    D. euphoria (6:I:1176)

Questions 213 to 217

Robert Jackson is an eighteen-year-old high school graduate who has come to the clinic for a health examination prior to employment. He lives with his widowed mother and a younger brother. He hopes to supplement his mother's income and take over some of the family responsibilities.

213. In doing the mental status assessment, the nurse would initially ask

    A. where Robert's father died
    B. for a spontaneous account of his life
    C. for an account of stressful factors in his life
    D. his present goals and how he hopes to meet these (20:149)

214. The nurse would expect that Robert would be involved in maturational tasks that relate to

    a. psychosexual identity
    b. personal autonomy and independence
    c. friendships
    d. reconciliation with practical reality

    A. a and d
    B. b and c
    C. c and d
    D. a, b, and c (20:154)

215. The nurse should recognize that Robert's ability to get a job and be financially independent is evidence that he has

    A. successfully accomplished the developmental task of his age
    B. began to make a vocational adaptation
    C. similar successful beginnings in heterosexual relationships
    D. the ability to function within groups (20:163)

216. Robert tells the nurse that his father died when he was four years old. The nurse will be particularly concerned with Robert's

    a. opportunity to identify with a male
    b. feelings of omnipotence
    c. relationship with his young brother
    d. feelings toward the opposite sex

    A. a and c
    B. b and d
    C. a, b, and c
    D. a and d (20:53–4)

217. Which of the following questions would elicit information regarding Robert's self-concept?

    a. What do you think about yourself?
    b. How do you think other people see you?
    c. What would you say about your mood?
    d. What do you imagine yourself doing in the future?

    A. a and b
    B. b and c
    C. a and c
    D. a, b, and d   (6:I:1168)

218. Which of the following is the most important objective of the initial interview?

    A. to begin the establishment of a therapeutic relationship
    B. to obtain essential data to identify current difficulties
    C. to evaluate motivation for treatment
    D. to explore present and past interpersonal and emotional difficulties
                              (18:547–48)

219. During the Mental Status Exam, the interviewer may need to be more active in order to accomplish which of the following goals?

    a. show interest in the client
    b. reduce the client's garrulity
    c. control irrelevance
    d. encourage the client's emotional expression

    A. a only
    B. a, b, and c
    C. b and d
    D. a, b, c, and d   (6:I:1147–51)

220. A patient's motivation for therapy and change can be assessed by considering data such as

    a. employment status
    b. dependency needs
    c. level of anxiety
    d. discomfort threshhold

    A. a and c
    B. b only
    C. c and d
    D. a, b, c, and d   (18:555)

221. Disturbances in ego function that indicate difficulty in the individual's ability to define reality and its relationship to self include

    a. identity confusion
    b. depersonalization
    c. hallucinations
    d. delusions

    A. a and c
    B. b, c, and d
    C. c and d
    D. a, b, c, and d   (18:553)

Directions: MATCH the following numbered items (behaviors) with the most appropriate lettered items (ego functions or dysfunctions).

Questions 222 to 231

222.	Cathexis	(4:18)
223.	Depersonalization	(4:28)
224.	Repetition compulsion	(4:84)
225.	Withdrawal	(4:101)
226.	Delusion	(4:27)
227.	Impulse disorder	(4:48)
228.	Bulimia	(4:16)
229.	Dreams	(21:259)
230.	Extreme narcissism	(4:61)
231.	Neologisms	(21:259)

    A. Reality perception or testing
    B. Object relations
    C. Regulation and control of drives
    D. Autistic thinking

Directions: For each of the following multiple choice questions, select the ONE most appropriate answer.

232. Which of the following characteristics is most important to assess in the first interview?

    A. depressive feeling
    B. sexual feelings
    C. motivation for treatment
    D. verbal ability   (18:552)

233. Which of the following symptoms are usually prompted by exogenous factors?

    a. illusions
    b. ideas of reference
    c. delusions
    d. hallucinations

    A. a and d
    B. a, b, and d
    C. b, c, and d
    D. a, b, and c   (4:47–8)

234. John Ryan, age 16, has been doing poorly in school and has been having trouble concentrating. The school nurse is talking with John and his mother in her office. Mrs. Ryan tells the nurse that John is an intelligent boy. The nurse asks John how he's been feeling. John answers that he feels sad. His mother interjects, "Of course, you're not sad. I'd know if you were sad. Now tell the nurse, you're just quiet." John replies, "I'm usually quiet, my mother is right." This is an example of

    A. double-bind
    B. mystification
    C. denial
    D. pseudomutuality   (6,I:189)

Questions 235 to 236

One day Miss Townsend seems in great distress and says to the nurse, "Can't somebody help me. There's electricity all over this place. Can't someone shut it off before it kills me?"

235. Miss Townsend is probably experiencing

    A. a delusion
    B. an hallucination
    C. an idea of reference
    D. an illusion   (20:105–06)

236. Which initial response to Miss Townsend indicates the best understanding of the nurse's role?

    A. "The electricity is not real. You must be experiencing a conflict."
    B. "I am not aware of any electricity here, but I can see that you are frightened."
    C. "I can see that you are upset. I'll make certain it's turned off."
    D. "You need to tell your doctor about this, Miss Townsend."   (34:200–02)

Directions: Each group of numbered words or phrases is followed by a list of lettered statements. MATCH the lettered statement most closely associated with the numbered word or phase.

Questions 237 to 241

237. Circumstantiality   (9:13)
238. Parapraxis   (4:68)
239. Perseveration   (20:104)
240. Blocking   (20:104)
241. Incoherence   (20:104)

    A. Speech has no logical order
    B. Expression and progression of thought suddenly cease
    C. Unable to distinguish essentials from nonessentials
    D. Clings to thoughts and repeats them
    E. Lapses of memory or blunders

Directions: For each of the following multiple choice questions, select the ONE most appropriate answer.

242. Retrograde amnesia refers to amnesia for events that occur

    A. after a significant point in time
    B. before a significant point in time
    C. as a result of organic causes
    D. as a result of emotional causes (20:120)

243. A boxer reports that after a blow on the head, he was unable to remember the rest of the fight even though he appeared normal. This is an example of

    A. retrograde amnesia
    B. anterograde amnesia
    C. paramnesia
    D. hypermnesia   (20:119)

244. When asked by the nurse if she had had visitors, Miss Stone replied, "My father came here and trees are growing in there, but the, I never can tell. Words, I get words from the voices." This is an example of

    A. flight of ideas
    B. ambivalence
    C. circumstantiality
    D. loosened association   (2:99)

245. Mrs. Lowery complains that she thinks that there are snakes inside her stomach. This is an example of

    A. a delusion
    B. an hallucination
    C. persecutory ideation
    D. hypochondriasis   (26:162)

246. The thought process, in which speech is rapid and with many sudden shifts of topics that remain comprehensible to others, is called

    A. an obession
    B. flight of ideas
    C. tangentiality
    D. circumstantiality   (21:498)

247. Which aspect of orientation is most fragile?

    A. time
    B. place
    C. person
    D. situation   (6:I:1169–79)

248. Miss Brown tells you that atomic rays are killing her family this very minute; she then laughs and gets up and starts dancing. This is an example of

    A. euphoria
    B. inappropriate affect

C. narcissism
D. circumstantiality   (10:232)

249. Which pair does *not* match?

    A. neologism—echolalia
    B. affect—feeling
    C. complex—hang-up
    D. amnesia—memory loss   (26:157–58)

250. On a windy night, Miss Wilson calls the nurse and insists that she hears someone coming up the stairway for her. The noises are obviously caused by the wind. Miss Wilson's behavior is most likely

    A. an illusion
    B. a delusion
    C. an hallucination
    D. false identification   (20:99)

251. Which statement best describes autistic thinking?

    A. it is controlled more by the thinker's needs or desires than by reality
    B. it is usually rational rather than irrational
    C. it is a necessary concomitant of creative thinking
    D. it achieves new solutions to problems and discovers new relationships (21:495)

252. A patient who overheard a radio in the next room said that this sound was the voice of her father. This is an example of a/an

    A. delusion
    B. auditory hallucination
    C. illusion
    D. idea of reference   (13:301)

253. A pregnant woman remarks to the nurse that she's so out of shape that she feels like a butterball. The nurse surmises that the client is exhibiting behavior related to her

    A. body image
    B. unresolved Electra complex
    C. denial of pregnancy
    D. ambivalence   (13:193)

254. The nurse is doing a mental status exam with an alert young woman who has had a history of anxiety attacks. The nurse might ask all of the following questions *except*

    A. "How are you feeling today"?
    B. "Tell me about your job."
    C. "Do you hear voices"?
    D. "What do you see as the difficulty"?
    (25:43)

255. Which of the following psychological tests are commonly used in diagnosing mental retardation?

    a. Stanford-Binet
    b. Rorschach
    c. M.M.P.I.
    d. Wechsler
    e. Bender-Gestalt

    A. a and b
    B. c
    C. a and d
    D. c and e
    (20:163–67)

256. Descriptive diagnoses are least useful in which of the following?

    A. insurance reports
    B. admission forms
    C. therapeutic plans
    D. epidemiological studies
    (2:91)

257. The American Psychiatric Association's Diagnostic and Statistical Manual of 1968 is

    A. identical to the International Classification of Diseases of the World Health Organization
    B. convertible to the World Health Organization's systems
    C. the first attempt by the U. S. to classify mental illness
    D. a system of classification based on the social model of mental disorder
    (6:I:1126)

258. For a nurse to correctly assess a client as being in a crisis state,

    a. the client must be aware of a sense of enormous difficulty
    b. the nurse must agree that the precipitating events are of crisis magnitude
    c. the client must have overt physical manifestations of crisis
    d. the client's usual coping mechanisms are not working for him

    A. a, b, and c
    B. b and c
    C. a and c
    D. a, b, c, and d
    (1:1–2)

259. In understanding the impact of illness upon the client's life, the "family" is defined as

    a. the primary family
    b. siblings, parents, and spouses
    c. those considered "significant" by the client
    d. the person cohabitating with the client

    A. a, b, c
    B. b, c, and d
    C. a, c, and d
    D. a, b, c, and d
    (30:112)

Directions: MATCH the numbered terms with the letter of the appropriate definition or example.

Questions 260 to 279

260.	Pathognomonic	(32:96)
261.	Confabulation	(10:410)
262.	Dyscontrol	(32:73)
263.	Double-bind	(30:197)
264.	Libido	(10:414)
265.	Autism	(10:410)
266.	Perseveration	(20:104)
267.	Projective identification	(32:93)
268.	Transference	(1:12)
269.	Dereism	(20:324)
270.	Security operations	(32:233)
271.	Pan anxiety	(20:337–38)
272.	Hobo syndrome	(20:330–31)
273.	Eclectic	(10:120)

274. Anhedonia (20:319)
275. Extinction (23:26)
276. Depersonalization (20:321)
277. Dissociation (20:81–2)
278. La Belle Indifference (20:419–20)
279. Cerea flexibilities (20:95–6)

A. Pseudoneurotic schizophrenia
B. Selecting from several systems
C. The tendency to falsify reality and to disregard realistic, logical, scientific thought
D. Feelings of vagueness, unreality, or detachment
E. Conversion hysteria
F. An abnormally persistent repetition or continuance in the expression of an idea
G. Psychic energy
H. The filling in of memory gaps with made up stories
I. An emotional reaction of the patient to the therapist in which the patient relives his conflicts and emotions as emerged from the unconscious past
J. Simple schizophrenia
K. Fugue state
L. The withholding of positive reinforcers following a response
M. An absorption in fantasy to the complete exclusion of reality
N. Characteristic or diagnostic of a specific disease
O. Lack of pleasure
P. Assumption that the other person is like you
Q. The way in which neurotics avoid natural experiencing in order to satisfy environmental demands
R. Suggestibility
S. Failure in coping
T. Damned if you do and damned if you don't

Chapter II: Answers and Explanations

1. **C.** Erikson, of the Institute of Human Development at Harvard, described the eight stages of man that represent a continuum from the beginning to the end of life.

2. **D.** Rather than evolving from a predetermined or preformed pattern (as in orthogenesis), this theory implies successive differentiation of an originally undifferentiated structure. For example, the eight stages of psychosocial development perceived by Erikson involve specific developmental tasks that must be solved in order to successfully proceed to subsequent phases.

3. **C.** These terms are to stress the fact that there are both positive and negative aspects present at each stage of development that are equally necessary.

4. **D.** According to Maslow, survival needs are basic followed by the need for security and safety. If these needs are fairly well met, the needs for love, affection, and belonging emerge, followed by esteem needs or discovery of self. Self-actualization or the desire for self-fulfillment is probably only met by about 1% of the population.

5. **D.** Vandenberg's study indicates that genetics influence numerical, spatial, verbal and word fluency, motor skills and personality factors of activity, vigor, impulsiveness, and sociability.

6. **D.** The behavioral patterns expressed by an adult are partially a reflection of how well he has completed the various developmental tasks. Each stage must be at least partially completed before the next is attempted.

7. **D.** Erikson's scheme takes account of the role that society and the individual himself play in the development of personality. The theory is basically an optimistic one, since each phase of growth has its strengths as well as its weaknesses. Thus failures at one stage can be rectified by successes at later stages.

8. **D.** These are examples of crises that occur in human beings. There is a threat or danger to life goals with tension and/or anxiety being experienced. Crises are turning points in which healthy or unhealthy adaptation can occur.

9. **C.** Each stage has a developmental time limit in which appropriate stimulation is needed in order to foster optimal development.

10. **B.** This is Piaget's preoperational stage. It starts with beginning of organized lauguage and is the period of greatest language growth.

11. **A.** The infant responds to an object only as long as it is directly available.

12. **C.** This is Piaget's concrete-operational stage. The child begins to try to communicate thoughts objectively and moves toward socialized speech.

13. **C.** A child still perceives right from wrong in a highly concrete and egocentric way but is beginning to make rational connections between cause and effect.

14. **D.** This is Piaget's stage of formal operations whereby the adolescent acquires the capacity to think and reason beyond his own realistic world and beliefs.

15. **B.** The child in the preoperational stage is unable to clearly distinguish between wish and reality.

16. **B.** The child can give a correct answer to a conceptual problem but cannot explain why this is so.

17. **A.** The infant learns to recognize that objects in the environment exist as separate and distinct from himself.

18. **C.** The child begins to use concepts of height and width in conservation.

19. **D.** The adolescent develops the ability to reason based on the logic of all possible combinations and controlled experimentation.

20. **A.** Research indicates that about fifty percent of a person's intellectual development occurs between conception and four years of age. About thirty percent takes place between ages four and eight.

21. **B.** Symbiosis refers to the relationship between two people who are totally dependent on each other, and therefore symbiosis is the opposite of independence. Likewise, isophilic and heterophilic are opposites. Isophilic refers to love of a person of the same sex whereas heterophilic refers to love of a person of the opposite sex.

22. **B.** The juvenile era (6 to 9 years of age) is associated with the tools of competition, compromise, and cooperation. These are utilized in tasks centering on peer relationships and learning.

23. **B.** These are tools of preadolescence. They are necessary for moving to a fully social state and for using learning to implement oneself for future life.

24. **C.** The collaborative relationship implies mutual influence.

25. **B.** Stress can precipitate anxiety which may range from mild anxiety to panic. Anxiety is differentiated from the similar response of fear by the fact that the stimulus is not related to a specific object.

26. **B.** There is an increase in perceptual abilities and an increased readiness to utilize cognitive abilities when a person is experiencing mild anxiety.

27. **D.** Some physiological responses such as muscle tension, perspiration, "butterflies" or headache may be present in moderate anxiety. However, in severe anxiety a person is likely to experience such sensations as nausea, trembling, dizziness, and feelings of dread, awe, or horror.

28. **C.** The ability of the person to develop more effective methods of adapting to stress also influence the prognosis.

29. **D.** During this terrifying experience the nurse needs to remind the client that she will stay with him. She should use short directive statements to help him feel that at least she is in control of the situation.

30. **D.** Alterations in the level of consciousness and self-awareness can be caused by such factors as direct injury to the brain or blood supply, metabolic dysfunctions, certain drugs, loss of a body part, decreased or disordered sensory stimulation, and anxiety.

31. **D.** A conflict is an antagonism between opposing forces and the level of consciousness can vary from fully conscious to fully unconscious.

32. **C.** Sensory deprivation produces hallucinations, mostly visual but some kinesthetic.

33. **D.** The components of alienation include social isolation, powerlessness, normlessness, meaninglessness, and self-estrangement. Alienation is the state of estrangement that one feels in cultural settings that he views as foreign, unpredictable, or unacceptable.

34. **A.** Roles held by individual family members tend to be influenced by the socioeconomic level of the family.

35. **A.** The ability to differentiate between the "me" and the "not me" is achieved through tactile experiences. Objects experienced through tactile communication like rattles, bottles, and mother are recognized quite early.

36. **B.** Social smiling begins between the second and eighth week and continues to about the twentieth week. It is evoked through visual presentation of various stimuli, most of them social in nature.

37. **A.** Eighth-month anxiety or "making strange" when the baby totally rejects strangers for his mother (even if she has been cold and unfeeling) tells us that he has learned to whom he belongs.

38. **D.** At age one year, the word mama is used in a wide variety of contexts; in another year or so it will be used appropriately.

39. **C.** Sometime between six to eight months, the infant develops the ability to differentiate his mother's face from those of other human beings. At this stage the infant finds the faces of others an unpleasant experience.

40. **A.** Primary prevention is aimed at providing some assurance that developmental needs of infants will be met.

41. **D.** Before the studies of Harlow, it was thought that the attachment was strictly a learned response with the reward being the gratifications which the infant received by having his needs met by his mother. This learning is part of the attachment process, but the studies of Harlow indicate that the infant is born with the capacity to emit attachment behavior toward the person caring for it.

42. **D.** The infant is born with the capacity to emit attachment behavior toward the person caring for it. These behaviors include clinging, vocalization, smiling, scanning and following.

43. **C.** Women who showed symptoms of crisis were those who seemingly denied the existence of any danger. They seemed to encourage a conspiracy of silence, avoiding any confrontation with feelings of fear, guilt, and anxiety.

44. **C.** The mother's chronic ignoring causes the infant to be overwhelmed and frantic. Thus he does not develop a sense of trust and develops undue fear each time he is separated and put down. Oversolicitous behavior never requires the infant to master the minimal stress of separation. Handling that is tense and jerky can cause anxiety and crying.

45. **B.** The oral needs of the infant are being severely frustrated. Painful tension is relieved by sucking and being helped.

46. **C.** An example of the types of disorders which one might classify as transient disturbances of infancy, are the symptomatic responses of the infant to separation from the mother.

47. **A.** If the individual, far beyond the age when the mouth should have ceased to be a focus of satisfaction, continues to be mouthcentered, he is said to be an oral type of personality. Egocentricity and dependency are examples of oral characteristics.

48. **D.** If the child has failed to speak by the end of three and one-half years (42 months) some problem invariably exists.

49. **D.** Autistic invention is the use of highly personal meanings for words and events. It is normally used by children. As the child grows and becomes socialized this process is replaced by consensual validation. If the child is cut off from replacing his autistic thoughts, thought disorders begin. Schizophrenia is a thinking disorder.

50. **B.** Almost all mothers in the study felt that a baby should know right from wrong by age 12 months. Mothers, who did not abuse their child, did not expect the child to be able to tell right from wrong before seven years of age.

51. **C.** Abusive mothers appear to have emotional difficulties, crying spells, feelings of isolation and loneliness, and poor interpersonal relationships with parents and friends. These women actively discourage friendships and do not join groups such as the PTA or local community group.

52. **B.** Upper-class mothers usually punished children for aggressive acts; middle-class mothers usually punished for activity, dangerous or otherwise; lower-class mothers punished for excessive demands, disobedience, and crying.

53. **D.** The child should be let know that he is in close association with an adult who will help and protect him. He should also be comforted by slight physical contact and by being held, once he is used to the nurse. The parents should be calmly informed that such cases have to be reported to appropriate authorities.

54. **D.** The stages are (1) protest, (2) despair, and (3) detachment. A, B, and C, describe the respective behaviors of these stages in sequence.

55. **B.** The trauma remains mild until the detachment phase. Once this phase is in progress the recovery will not be without residual emotional scarring.

56. **D.** The chances are ninety-nine percent that the enuresis is caused by emotional tension. Since urinalysis generally screens out both physical disease and anatomic abnormality, cystoscopy and an elaborate work-up of the urinary tract are not crucial. These procedures often frighten the child.

57. **C.** It is a normal curiosity for 3 to 5 year olds, and direct observation is the only means for satisfying it. If the child is allowed to observe the differences at toilet time, the interest should subside before the child starts school. The nurse accepts the behavior of the children as a normal curiosity typical of their developmental stage.

58. **C.** Regression is a process in which the personality reverses developmental steps, moving backward to earlier interests, defenses, and modes of gratification.

59. **D.** In this case the problem is one of sibling rivalry. Paul needs to be reassured of his continued secure position in the family. Attention would help to give him this feeling.

60. **D.** Johnny is in the Oedipal Stage of development and thus nightmares arise even in well-adjusted children. The parents may not fully understand the developmental aspects of anxiety. If Johnny's nightmares are frequent, one might suspect neurotic problems with a need for psychotherapy.

61. **A.** As Johnny is in the Oedipal Phase of development, his nightmares may be symbolic of his wishes to usurp father's place. His success in occupying father's place may add to this conflict.

62. **D.** This technique would present Johnny with the reality of a secure mother-father bond which would meet his needs and strengthen his sense of security in the family.

63. **A.** During this period, the child's use of language and locomotion permits him to expand his

imagination. Intrusive behaviors include aggressive talking.

64. **B.** The child from four to eight years of age has intense curiosity about human sexuality. The child may explore, with considerable candor, or show concern for the genitals of both sexes.

65. **C.** A child with a school phobia exhibits severe anxiety, dread and apprehension, and psychosomatic complaints associated almost exclusively with the necessity to attend school. On weekends and during vacation periods, the symptoms usually disappear in a matter of hours, only to reappear when school attendance is anticipated or forced.

66. **D.** Children with school phobias are usually of average or above average intelligence; they respect authority, and are from an achievement-oriented home environment.

67. **C.** Treatment consists of returning the child to school as soon as possible and helping the family to allow the child more autonomy.

68. **B.** The underlying psychopathology is believed to be an intense separation anxiety rooted in unresolved dependency ties.

69. **B.** In children after the age of ten, phobias have more complex roots and merit psychiatric evaluation.

70. **A.** Social accommodation arises from the child's experience with his compeers. Social subordination occurs as a result of the juvenile's experiences with authority figures other than his parents.

71. **B.** Excessive rebelliousness may arise from either overpermissiveness or overcontrolling behavior on the part of the parents and will lead to the child's not learning to share and cooperate in social situations.

72. **D.** Stealing represents a conduct disturbance of childhood.

73. **C.** Freud considered that phobias are, par excellence, the neuroses of childhood.

74. **C.** Short periods of regressive messiness and obstinancy, arrogance, and grandiosity are usually transient disorders and represent a normal phase of development. In part, they express the need of the adolescent to individuate and his groping attempts to do so.

75. **D.** The fifth stage of psychosocial development, Identity and Repudiation vs. Identity Diffusion, occurs between 12 and 18 years of age. Erikson believes that the ultimate goal of the individual at this time is to acquire a sense of identity, which is never gained nor maintained once and for all.

76. **D.** Components of a sense of identity are: (1) a feeling of being at home in one's body, (2) a sense of "knowing where one is going," (3) an inner certainty of anticipated recognition from those who count, and (4) a readiness to face the challenges of the adult world. Kohlberg believes that the person, having completed adolescence, has a new awareness of the world, and values the awareness of new meanings in life.

77. **B.** When an individual does not come to grips with the question of who he is, he suffers from self-diffusion. The adolescent frequently overidentifies with other adolescents or groups, attempting to take on their values, ideals or appearance. The central task of adolescence is that of identity versus self-diffusion.

78. **C.** Some clinicians view normal adolescent turmoil as resembling borderline psychopathology. Although this notion persists in the thinking of many clinicians, recent data indicate that adolescent turmoil reflects psychopathology rather than normal development and that turmoil is an infrequent phenomenon. Emotional conflicts seen as normal adolescent turmoil by one investigator may be viewed as pathological by another.

79. **C.** According to Erikson, the central concern of the young adult is Intimacy and Solidarity vs. Isolation.

80. **C.** In early adulthood, there is an increasing concern with one's work or vocation.

81. **D.** Based upon results of current research, all four items are sexual myths.

82. **C.** Some degree of fatigue, irritability, and low spirits is present in women when conception has not occurred following ovulation. Hormone production abruptly drops to almost zero about 12 days after ovulation.

83. **B.** Havighurst's tasks of early adulthood include the taking on of civic responsibility.

84. **B.** Miss Bush is in the stage of young adulthood. According to Erikson, the central conflict of this stage of life is that of intimacy and solidarity vs. isolation. The sexual and psychological intimacies that two people have in a love relationship may be viewed as very threatening.

85. **D.** In order to escape anxiety or conflict, the defense mechanism of avoidance is commonly used. In this case, Miss Bush avoids the anxiety by focusing on the present rather than on future plans.

86. **A.** The largest proportion of divorces occur in the early years of marriage among childless couples.

87. **A.** Divorces are more common among marriages with urban background, early marriage (15 to 19 years), short courtship and/or short engagement, mixed race or religion, disapproval of friends, and relatives, dissimilar backgrounds, and unhappy parental marriages.

88. **C.** It seems apparent that unresolved neurotic patterns influence mate selection. These patterns, carried over from one marriage to another, tend to reinforce one's failure pattern in the subsequ marriage.

89. **B.** The peak period of divorces is in the second year of marriage, after which the rate drops rapidly.

90. **B.** It is not uncommon for a person faced with a loss to express anger at the person who relays the bad news.

91. **A.** Viewing of the corpse helps to establish the reality of death, a necessary step in the process of mourning.

92. **E.** In order for recovery to take place, feelings must be detached from the lost object with a reorganization of behavior directed toward a new object. Sometimes there is a brief frenetic phase of reaching out in search of a new object.

93. **A.** The initial reaction to loss is frequently shock and disbelief.

94. **D.** Feelings of despair are often accompanied by withdrawal, regression, and disorganization.

95. **C.** This represents the cry for help. The prototype of this is the infant who, when missing the mother, cries and the mother returns.

96. **E.** Remarriage may indicate the mourner has completed his grief work and is ready to seek out new relationships.

97. **C.** What is wanted is assistance in reunion, a need to right the wrong, the instinct that all losses are retrievable.

98. **B.** The involutional period is that which occurs during menopause.

99. **B.** Transient situational behavior reactions appear to be acute and temporary responses to emotionally distressing, depriving, or fearful situations.

100. **D.** The basic task of old age is the "acceptance of one's own life cycle." Fear of death results from a sense of despair at what might have been, and the feeling that life is too short to start again and reach this sense of integrity by an alternate route.

101. **B.** Contact and exchange between parents and children is usually desired but on a limited basis—for example, frequent visiting rather than living in the same household.

102. **C.** This theory of disengagement was developed by Cumming and Henry in systematically explaining human aging as a social-psychological phenomena.

103. **D.** The basic theme of this phase is rooted in the interest in establishing and guiding the next generation. Obviously maturity can be attained at this level without the actual parenting of children.

104. **D.** It is now clearly established to be a universal mental process of aging. The life review is not relegated solely to the years of later maturity but can come at times of stress and threat, such as impending death, during earlier years.

105. **A.** The normative crisis of the middle years is "the crisis of generativity which occurs when a man looks at what he has generated or helped to generate and finds it good or wanting." Stagnation results when the individual turns inward and becomes self-absorbed and "indulges himself as if he were his one and only child."

106. **B.** Aging increases the susceptibility to illness and the probability of death.

107. **B.** George Maddox has shown that elderly people are more objective and open about their health if they have had extensive contact with others their own age.

108. **C.** Although we may conceive of aging in terms of decline, this decline is a movement toward a final end.

109. **C.** There are frequent misconceptions about the aged. Only about 5% of the aged reside in institutions. Although people often tend to infantilize older persons, ability and intelligence remain relatively intact providing no major illness develops. In the absence of illness, sexual activity can be maintained into the 70's and 80's.

110. **B.** With a decrease in the sense of taste, there is a decrease in the sense of smell. Older people frequently have loss of teeth and problems with dentures.

111. **D.** Hearing loss in the aged is especially acute for high frequencies; thus men have a worse time than women.

112. **D.** Although there are evident changes in terms of tendency to learn, there is little evidence of change in learning capacity.

113. **C.** Cumming and Henry have developed a rather systematic explanation of human aging as a social-psychological phenomenon. This theory conceives the aging individual as being at the center of a network of social interactions. As he ages, his life space tends to constrict and he curtails his social life.

114. **C.** Psychic determinism, based on the principle of causality, is the theoretical foundation of psychotherapy and psychoanalysis.

115. **C.** Each type of physical illness has special meanings and poses problems to the sick person. Short-term modifications of his behavior are seen as coping processes, whereas long-term modifications are usually viewed as adaptive.

116. **D.** Anxiety is a subjectively experienced emotion which is characterized by feelings of vague, unexplained discomfort and apprehension. However, a person's perceptive abilities are increased, as is his learning ability, with a mild degree of anxiety.

117. **D.** *Ambivalence* is the existence within the person of opposing emotions, impulses, or desires. *Trauma* is an experience that inflicts serious damage upon the person. It often results in maladjusted (conflicted) behavior. *Stress* is any physical or psychological force that, when applied to a system is sufficient to cause strain or distortion in the system, or when very great, to alter the system. The person is then required to change in some way. This may pose a conflict between the status quo and the new behavior.

118. **D.** Cultural and psychological factors, both conscious and unconscious, are of considerable importance. For example, with food, we all become hungry in the same way but the list of materials that one person or one group considers as food may differ from that of another person or group.

119. **D.** For normal development of the personality, the ego must be able to modify both the id drives and the superego's demands for acceptable conduct without extreme sacrifice of either emotional and instinctive satisfaction or of ethical ideals. Ego functions are guided by reality principles. Through reason and circumspection, they deal rationally with the requirements of reality and of society when the ego is said to be strong and healthy.

120. **A.** It is often a matter of considerable significance in prognosis and therapy to determine whether a patient's emotional illness is primarily a matter of regression or of fixation. It is almost always easier to help a patient regain a level of maturity that he has once before achieved than it is to help him attain such a level for the first time.

121. **B.** Symptoms that are ego syntonic are less likely to motivate change because change in intensive therapy means more work for the ego.

122. **B.** Strong, unconscious ambivalent feelings may play important roles in causing psychiatric disorders. A large part of psychiatric treatment is devoted to helping people become aware of and comfortable with their ambivalent feelings. Ambivalence occurs to some extent in all close interpersonal relationships.

123. **A.** When the forces of the id threaten to overwhelm the ego, the ego brings into action defense mechanisms which are manifested behaviorally as symptoms.

124. **C.** Frustrations of all kinds which increase the anxiety and tension under which we live are experienced in our complex society.

125. **C.** Fixation is used to describe the condition in which the intellectual and physical aspects of development have continued, but the sexual-social drives have retained the aims and the objects of an early period of life.

126. **D.** Anxiety can cause one to have distorted perceptions as can fatigue, intoxication, and lack of sensory stimulation. All these factors can induce a person to misinterpret objects. For example, fatigue from driving on a long, monotonous road can provoke illusions of obstacles in the road.

127. **A.** The ego defense mechanisms are internal mechanisms of control, unconsciously selected and operating automatically. They are designed to manage anxiety, aggressive impulses, hostilities, resentments and frustrations. They are not necessarily pathological.

128. **C.** This mechanism derives its name from the word "introject" which literally means to take into or ingest. One incorporates and accepts attitudes of others.

129. **D.** In displacement, the unacceptable feeling is transferred to a safer substitute object.

130. **C.** Depressed patients utilize the mechanism of introjection; the anger is turned inward. In projection, the anger would be expressed outwardly.

131. **C.** Rationalization occurs when an individual substitutes another reason for the real reason motivating his behavior.

132. **B.** Conversion is an unconscious process by which an emotional conflict is expressed as a physical symptom. In this case, the anxiety about completing the term paper is handled by the fact her hand becomes immobilized.

133. **C.** Identification involves the taking on of selected aspects of a significant other, whereas introjection occurs at a much earlier phase of development from which evolve "good" or "bad" images of the self. Incorporation takes place when the mourning process is not successfully negotiated due to unresolved feelings of hostility to the lost object. Empathy is a healthy form of identification which is limited and temporary—the capacity for projecting oneself into the situation and feelings of others.

134. **D.** The explanation given may indeed be true but it is not *the* reason.

135. **C.** One method of handling anxiety is to behave in a manner exactly opposite of what the person is actually feeling. This unconscious defense is called reaction formation. If a person consciously behaved in this manner, we would say he was a hyprocrite.

136. **C.** Denial is a defense mechanism by means of which consciously intolerable thoughts, wishes, facts, and deeds are disowned by an unconscious denial of their existence. What is consciously intolerable is unconsciously rejected by a protective mechanism of nonawareness. Denial is not the same as malingering or lying.

137. **D.** Reaction formation is a defense mechanism, operating unconsciously, wherein attitudes and behavior are adopted that are the opposites of impulses the individual harbors unconsciously.

138. **C.** In displacement, an emotional feeling is transferred from its actual object to a substitute. The feeling originally directed toward a certain person, object, or situation is transferred to another person, object, or situation.

139. **C.** Suppression is a conscious effort made to dismiss repudiated strivings and undesired memories from awareness.

140. **F.** Sublimation is the release into a different situation of the unused energy or impulses which cannot be realized or socially approved in one situation.

141. **B.** Conversion is a mechanism whereby an individual converts an emotional problem into a physical symptom.

142. **I.** In reaction formation, unconscious desires and attitudes may be repressed and replaced by the adoption of conscious attitudes which are the opposite of the unconscious ones.

143. **E.** Displacement is a transfer into another situation of an emotion felt in a previous situation where its expression would not have been socially acceptable.

144. **J.** Symbolism is a mechanism whereby a person attaches significance to shapes of objects, colors, slogans, and words.

145. **D.** Condensation is the fusion of two or more ideas or experiences into one experience or manifestation.

146. **A.** Suppression is the conscious, deliberate forcing of unpleasant anxiety—producing experiences into the unconscious mind.

147. **G.** Denial is the mechanism of ignoring or refusing to acknowledge the existence of unpleasant or disagreeable realities of living.

148. **C.** Undoing is an unconscious, symbolic attempt to eradicate or eliminate the existence of a previous painful experience.

149. **H.** Rationalization is a defense which explains and justifies an individual's ideas, actions, and feelings in a plausible light.

150. **C.** This symbolic act serves as a sort of magic ritual by which he undoes or annuls the possible effect of his unrecognized impulses and achieves atonement.

151. **D.** Identification is a defense mechanism, operating unconsciously, by which an individual endeavors to pattern himself after another. Identification plays a major role in the development of one's personality and specifically of one's superego.

152. **B.** This is a primitive defense mechanism, operating unconsciously, in which something unacceptable and already done is symbolically acted out in reverse, usually repetitiously, in the hope of "undoing" it and thus relieving anxiety.

153. **C.** This defense mechanism, operates unconsciously, whereby that which is emotionally unacceptable in the self is unconsciously rejected and attributed to others.

154. **B.** By preconscious is meant all mental activity of which one is not aware but which can be brought into awareness with effort.

155. **A.** Sublimation is a technique through which the libidinal drive is deflected into other channels of discharge, channels affording sufficient release of

tension for the individual to remain in a state of adjustment.

156. **A.** One quite reliable clue to the existence of transference factors in a relationship has to do with the rapidity with which one's attitudes toward the other person takes form. "Love at first sight" before one has had the opportunity to get to know the recipient of the feeling, is almost invariably strongly influenced by unrecognized transference factors.

157. **C.** Reversal is the technique whereby an instinctive impulse is seemingly turned into its opposite.

158. **A.** In reversal, an instinctual impulse is seemingly turned into its opposite. Thus it differs from reaction formation in that the latter involves a thoroughgoing change in attitude, where reversal involves an action or a manifestation of an impulse.

159. **C.** Projection is a technique whereby feelings, wishes, or attitudes originating within the subject are attributed by him to persons or other objects in his environment.

160. **C.** This is a mechanism used to evade or escape unpleasant or disagreeable realities of living by ignoring or refusing to acknowledge their existence.

161. **D.** They may be viewed as reactions to conflict which are associated with one of the three major defense patterns: moving against, moving away, and moving toward.

162. **B.** Reaction formation is another term for overcompensation.

163. **B.** Regression is something that happens to the personality, whereas other defense mechanisms are generally functions of the ego.

164. **B.** Taking on socially undesirable characteristics, if these appear to provide some special strength, is sometimes referred to, in particular, as hostile identification.

165. **A.** Difficulties related to making plans are observed with loneliness. There is a vacillation between overplanning and planlessness.

166. **D.** The client may use all these behaviors. In idealizing others, the client may invest the nurse with all the potential qualities for meeting his unmet wishes and needs. Role-reversal can be seen as a way that the client tests if the nurse's needs supercede his own. Somatic participation is a way of relating based on the expression of bodily needs. It's easier to talk about the strength one lacks than to talk about the weakness one feels. Peplau identifies these three "attitudes" as common ways that clients attempt to establish contact.

167. **C.** The actual mechanism whereby identification is brought about is introjection. Imitation is a conscious process. Identification is unconscious.

168. **C.** The fact that certain ideas assume a delusional intensity is evidence of the severe regression that has taken place making reality-testing inadequate.

169. **D.** Regression is something that happens to the personality; the ego does not actively bring it about.

170. **C.** There are some homosexuals whose ego functioning otherwise appears intact and who conduct themselves both effectively and constructively in society.

171. **B.** The psychiatric history focuses on the content of individual experience and therefore is more subjective. If the nurse is a skillful interviewer, a wealth of data can be obtained from a good history.

172. **D.** Interjecting a proverb at an inappropriate time and in an inappropriately loud voice most likely speaks for a schizophrenic process. Answer C may represent the meaning of this highly symbolic communication but we cannot be sure at this point.

173. **D.** The nurse herself is an essential measuring instrument since proper timing, explanation, and emphasis on the positive value of certain tests are necessary to enlist cooperation.

174. **A.** The impressionistic aspect of the MSE is collected during the history taking, while the psychometric or explicit cognitive testing is usually done later.

175. **B.** Kinetics refers to motion rather than appearance.

176. **D.** This is an example of feeling that events in the environment are of specific personal significance. The idea is not delusional since it is not a fixed idea and it is not necessarily persecutory in nature.

177. **A.** A person of average intelligence should be able to see objects and concepts in terms of "abstract or general classes."

178. **B.** Fewer than 5 adequate responses suggests below average intellectual functioning, 5 to 8 correct responses is average and more than 8 correct responses is above average.

179. **D.** Cognitive tests are useful for all three reasons. Changes over time are important for differentiating delirium from dementia and for gauging the effect of anxiety on thought processes.

180. **D.** Serial subtraction is one of the most valuable tests in detecting slight changes in attention. Long before arithmetical error may occur, the patient may betray his decreasing ability to perform the task by heightened effort, perseveration, increase in total time needed, frequent hesitation or questioning, requesting a new start, or becoming irritable or by deprecating the test and the examiner.

181. **C.** Average time for serial 7 subtraction is up to 90 seconds. Four or more errors is considered marginal and 7 or more errors is considered quite poor performance.

182. **D.** It is desirable to offer the least amount of structure that will enable the patient to communicate.

183. **C.** The process of the interview refers to the developing relationship between therapist and patient. It is particularly concerned with the implicit meaning of the communication. It includes the manner in which the patient and therapist relate to each other.

184. **D.** The Rorschach test tells much about the patient's feelings, emotional turmoil and personality structure. The TAT allows the patient to project his feelings, daydreams, experiences, and emotional conflicts. The Sentence Completion test searches the patient's attitudes and feelings in many areas of his life. The Draw-a-Person test allows for speculation on the patient's basic attitudes toward persons of both sexes and toward his mother and his father.

185. **B.** Direct questions are used only after other approaches have been tried, unless the client seems obviously disoriented.

186. **D.** Insight refers to the client's understanding of his illness and the attendant circumstance.

187. **D.** Different experiences give different meanings to outwardly similar events. The interviewer always seeks to leave the meaning of the event for the client.

188. **B.** The purpose of the Mental Status Examination is to provide an accurate description of the patient's current functioning. The record can be used as a base line for later comparisons.

189. **C.** While the quality of the client's fantasy life is part of the "thought content," so are his dreams, ambitions, fears, and identifications.

190. **D.** One's psychological state can vary widely with changes in the external environment.

191. **C.** The therapist cannot expect to promote healing without awareness of these assets. One needs to help the client utilize his strengths.

192. **C.** Many symptoms have adaptive or defensive value, others do not. Therefore it is inaccurate to view symptoms solely as defensive mechanisms.

193. **C.** It is important to know if a person is correctly oriented in all three spheres - time, place and person. Being more than three days off as to the date is highly suspicious of disorientation.

194. **B.** An impression of distractability can be obtained by casually dropping a pencil or glancing at one's watch to see if such minor stimuli disrupt the patient's ongoing behavior.

195. **D.** Both recent and past memory can be tested during the regular history taking. Recent memory may be tested by asking the person to recall your name, his route to the hospital, a recent meal, etc.

196. **F.** A patient's fund of information and vocabulary are the two best indicators of his general level of intelligence. They are particularly useful because of their relative insensitivity to the effects of any but the relatively most severe forms of psychopathology.

197. **G.** Patients must be able to give a reasonable definition or in any other way indicate their understanding of the *meaning* of the word.

198. **A.** The patient's capacity for abstraction—the ability to generalize, to think in terms of classes of objects and of events and to understand the meaning and implication of symbols—is frequently tested by the use of proverbs or similarities.

199. **E.** When assessing intellectual function, it is important to find out the extent to which the patient has been able to acquire an understanding of common modes of behavior in society and an understanding of common social mores and conventions.

200. **H.** In order to test for a person's perceptual and motor functioning, you can ask him to write his name or copy a simple geometric figure on a sheet of blank paper.

201. **A.** The history includes important areas of life experience and often provides major clues to the psychodynamic factors influencing the illness and its progress.

202. **D.** Although varying in emphasis and detail with different patients, some psychiatric assessment should form part of every careful health assessment.

203. **B.** The data will be incomplete even if the interviewer spends several sessions, as the patient may withhold information. Therefore any clinical impressions are tentative formulations.

204. **B.** In providing initial structure, the less organized the patient's current ego-functioning, the more structure the interviewer must provide.

205. **C.** It is important that the interviewer note the general appearance, manner and attitude of the client and be alert to any peculiarities or incongruities present.

206. **B.** Disturbances in the regulation of drives are seen in acting out behavior.

207. **A.** Depersonalization and an unstable body image are examples of problems with reality relationships.

208. **E.** This indicates compulsive behavior and the use of undoing.

209. **D.** Paranoid thinking is a type of disturbed thought process.

210. **C.** This indicates an excessive closeness with another.

211. **B.** A delusion is a false belief. Hallucinations and illusions are disorders of perception. Ambivalence has to do with opposing drives.

212. **B.** Depersonalization is a loss of feeling of personal identity with one's self.

213. **B.** A patient's spontaneous account of himself will usually expose more informative material than the patient realizes.

214. **D.** Adolescence is a period of emerging personal identity with struggles for autonomy and independence.

215. **B.** It is important to recognize that the individual's emotional development may not have advanced equally in all respects or in all relationships.

216. **D.** When the Oedipus complex is inadequately resolved, the individual may introject some of the qualities of the parent of the opposite sex and thus preclude normal relationships with persons of the opposite sex.

217. **D.** The set of thoughts that the client entertains about himself constitutes his self-concept.

218. **A.** The initial contact between therapist and patient has been identified as having great bearing on the development of the therapeutic relationship which is the ultimate aim of a therapeutic interview. The others are important purposes that enable one to maintain a therapeutic relationship.

219. **D.** The examiner should express, by word or gesture, some understanding of the patient's problems and his appreciation for his cooperation. The right of the client to say what he wants, does not convey the right to ramble on tediously.

220. **D.** Assessment of motivation includes the consideration of external factors (loss of job), degree of dependency needs, the amount of discomfort the person is experiencing, and his capacity to tolerate discomfort while in therapy.

221. **D.** Disturbances in this sphere may be seen in the adoption of rigid roles, delusions, hallucinations, denial, depersonalization, identity confusion, and an unstable body image.

222. **B.** Cathexis is attachment of emotional feeling and significance to an idea or object, most commonly a person.

223. **A.** Depersonalization refers to feelings of unreality concerning the environment, the self, or both.

224. **C.** Repetition compulsion is the impulse to reenact earlier emotional experiences. The impulse is carried out quite irrespective of any advantage that doing so might bring from a pleasure-pain point of view.

225. **B.** Withdrawal is a pathological retreat from people or the world of reality.

226. **A.** A delusion is a false belief out of keeping with the individual's level of knowledge and his cultural group.

227. **C.** Impulse disorder refers to disorders in which impulse control is weak.

228. **C.** Bulimia is morbidly increased hunger.

229. **D.** Autistic thinking is frequently found in dreams. Objective considerations such as time and place, possible and impossible, have little weight.

230. **B.** Narcissism is self-love as opposed to object love. In excess, it interferes with relations with others.

231. **D.** Neologisms are newly coined words that are not primarily used in the service of communication but rather in the service of self-expression.

232. **A.** In the first interview, one should assess current functioning by noting any signs of depression and asking the client whether he is subject to depression and therefore a suicide risk.

233. **D.** Ideas of reference are the incorrect interpretations of casual incidents and external events as having direct reference to one's self. An illusion is the misinterpretation of a real experience.

234. **B.** Mystification is a process in which the person is systematically forced to deny data from one realm in the interest of maintaining a percept or relationship.

235. **A.** The threat of unworthy desires or of troublesome and disowned aspects of the personality are projected as hostility from the environment.

236. **B.** The nurse tells the patient she does not agree with her while telling her she realizes that her feelings are real.

237. **C.** In circumstantiality, the person proceeds indirectly to his goal idea, giving many tedious details and irrelevant additions.

238. **E.** A faulty act, blunder, or lapse of memory such as a slip of the tongue, constitute parapraxis. According to Freud, these acts are unconsciously motivated.

239. **D.** Perseveration is the abnormally persistent repetition or continuance in expression of an idea.

240. **B.** In blocking, both expression and progression of thought suddenly cease. Blocking to a severe degree seems to be confined to schizophrenia.

241. **A.** The progress of thinking is so disorderly that one idea runs into another without logical consecution and speech is not bound by any law. Scattered thinking is similar but a little less disorderly.

242. **B.** In retrograde amnesia, there is a loss of memory extending back over a period of time prior to the time when the onset occurred.

243. **B.** Anterograde amnesia is one that extends forward to cover a period following the apparent regaining of environmental contact.

244. **D.** Loosened association is a form of fragmentation of thought. Thought processes lose their smooth continuity and may be difficult to follow.

245. **A.** This is a somatic delusion. The client thinks this is so, which implies a false belief motivated by the affective aspect of the personality.

246. **B.** Flight of ideas is a morbid type of thought sequence manifested through speech, characterized by its rapidity and by numerous and sudden shifts in topics, but which tends to be comprehensible to the normal observer.

247. **A.** The sense of time seems to be the first to become disorganized as organic brain syndromes develop.

248. **B.** The emotional response to what the person is saying does not match and is therefore inappropriate.

249. **A.** Echolalia is repeating the speech of another. Neologism is the coining of new words that have symbolic meaning.

250. **A.** A perceptional misinterpretation is known as an illusion.

251. **A.** Thought processes are determined by inner needs and relatively uninfluenced by environmental considerations.

252. **C.** This is an example of a mistaken sensory perception. The client misidentifies the sound.

253. **A.** The client's conscious and unconscious image may differ from each other. She may think of her body as it was before and long for its return.

254. **C.** One does not ask an obviously non-psychotic patient if he hears voices. One asks questions that appear appropriate and are based on one's observation of the patient.

255. **C.** Intelligence is assessed through the Stanford-Binet Intelligence Scale and the Wechsler Intelligence Scale. The Rorschach is a projective test that assesses personality characteristics and underlying dynamics, and the Bender-Gestalt, a drawing test, is now primarily used as a general projective technique. Important phases of personality and personality adaptation are examined on the Minnesota Multiphasic Personality Inventory.

256. **C.** The descriptive diagnosis is used for hospital admission and discharge forms, insurance reports, and other administrative purposes, but much more information is required to understand a patient.

257. **B.** Changes were adopted in 1968 to make the APA system compatible with that of the WHO's system and interconvertible with it.

258. **C.** A person in crisis faces a problem that he cannot readily solve by using the coping mechanisms that have worked for him before. Although the problem may seem minor to the nurse, the person in crisis feels helpless and thus has a rise of inner tension and anxiety.

259. **D.** Usually, a family is a small group of people tied together by a legal arrangement, sex and/or love, heredity, common goals and/or customs and/or beliefs. Since at times few of these elements are present, it is usually best to view as the "family" any group of people who consider themselves to be one.

260. **N.** For example, "almost pathognomic" symptoms of schizophrenia include audible thoughts, voices conversing with one another and delusional perceptions.

261. **H.** These made-up stories that the patient believes to be true are common to organic psychoses.

262. **S.** This is a concept described by Menninger having to do with the disruption of thought processes, confusion, and escape of disruptive impulses. It greatly increases the potential for violence.

263. **R.** This type of interaction is generally associated with schizophrenic families. One person demands a response to a message containing mutually contradictory signals while the other is unable to respond or comment on the inconsistent and incongruous message.

264. **G.** This is a psychoanalytic term meaning vital force.

265. **M.** Examples of autistic behavior are hallucinations and day dreams.

266. **F.** This clinging to the same thought is frequently seen in aphasia, catatonia, and in those with senile dementia.

267. **O.** This is the forerunner to ideas of reference and influence.

268. **I.** The patient transfers to the therapist emotions that he had felt toward authority figures in his childhood.

269. **C.** This type of primary process thinking is not corrected by the logic of experiences or by the demands of the environment.

270. **Q.** These activities are required for reduction or relief of tension in order to maintain a feeling of safety in another's esteem.

271. **A.** This kind of diffuse anxiety pervades all the patient's life experiences and although he tries to force pleasurable experiences, he does not derive pleasure from anything. This type of anxiety is seen in pseudo-neurotic schizophrenia—an underlying schizophrenic disorder hidden by a facade of neurotic manifestations.

272. **J.** The simple schizophrenic is frequently an irresponsible idler, vagrant, tramp, prostitute, or delinquent.

273. **B.** An eclectic approach is one which draws from a number of theories or schools of thought.

274. **O.** The anhedonic derives little pleasure or satisfaction from his accomplishments. This state is common to the schizophrenic process.

275. **L.** When a mother responds to a child's temper tantrums by leaving the room, she is using extinction.

276. **D.** A person experiencing feelings of depersonalization frequently complains of being a spectator in life rather than taking part in it.

277. **K.** This kind of psychological separation or splitting off serves as an intrapsychic defensive process which operates automatically and unconsciously in the face of painful anxiety. Amnesia, fugue state, and multiple personality are all examples of dissociation.

278. **E.** This pathological tranquility is of diagnostic significance in a conversion reaction. The conflict has been solved through denial and the anxiety has been relieved by the conversion of the repressed impulses and wishes into a functional system.

279. **R.** Cerea flexibilitas or waxy flexibility is a form of immobility seen in catatonics. When the joints of the patient's extremities are flexed or extended with a wax-like rigidity, the patient retains the position imposed much like the limbs of a jointed doll.

CHAPTER III

Psychopathology and Nursing Intervention

INTRODUCTION

The focus of this chapter will be psychiatric disorders and their nursing care. The standard diagnostic nomenclature will be utilized, as it is the belief of the authors that professional nurses need to know and understand this classification system in order to participate as equals on the psychiatric team. The authors recognize the limitations of this system as it is largely a descriptive one. Thus the dynamics of the disorders will be emphasized as the basis for appropriate nursing intervention. It is the meaning of the behavior that is the focus of nursing intervention. Only through understanding the client's life experience and relating it to psychodynamic theory can the nurse provide the client with experiences that will promote healthy behavior. The nurse acquires this understanding through the professional relationship with its content, mood and interaction themes. While general principles of nursing intervention can be identified, specific responses may vary according to the personalities of the nurse and the client.

Situations will be presented throughout the chapter and the authors recognize that disagreement may exist regarding appropriate intervention. We have attempted to clearly define the situations to keep this disagreement to a minimum but we recognize that other theorists may find another alternative more sound from their particular viewpoint. An eclectic approach is presented and attention will be given to several models and theories. The predominant models are the medical, social, psychological and behavioral ones: the theories are Freudian or Sullivanian. Certain theories and models lend themselves to particular psychiatric disorders. For example, the social model is frequently seen as most suitable for working with the alcoholic, whereas, the medical model might be most suited for the understanding and treatment of a patient with an endogenous depression. Issues involving dynamics and treatment remain a fact of life in the field of psychiatric nursing and are the basis of current research.

A.   Neuroses

Directions: For each of the following multiple choice questions, select the ONE most appropriate answer.

1.   Neurotic behavior is best described as behavior that demonstrates the

A.   loss of the ability to adapt
B.   inability to feel subjective psychic pain
C.   lack of either primary or secondary gains
D.   presence of subjectively distressing behavior   (4:63)

60

2. Neurotic behavior is distinguished from psychotic behavior by

   a. the patient's awareness of a disturbance
   b. the absence of gross reality distortion
   c. the lack of subjective anxiety
   d. symptoms that are ego alien

   A. a and b
   B. b and c
   C. a, b, and c
   D. a, b, and d   (10:205)

3. Neurotic symptoms are

   A. ego alien
   B. ego syntonic
   C. ego disintegrative
   D. all of the above   (10:205)

4. Which of the psychoneuroses illustrates the most severe psychopathology?

   A. obsessive compulsive type
   B. conversion type
   C. hypochondriacal type
   D. dissociative type   (21:165)

5. The typical psychoneurosis does not require

   A. severe external stress
   B. predisposing factors
   C. ego impairment
   D. forbidden impulses   (21:141)

6. Which theorist hypothesized that the psychoneurotic patient suffers from basic anxiety, that is, a feeling of intrinsic weakness and helplessness toward a world perceived as hostile and dangerous?

   A. Frieda Fromm-Reichmann
   B. Anna Freud
   C. Karen Horney
   D. Erich Fromm   (18:339)

7. A man has a recurring thought that he may jump off a high place or out of a moving car. His behavior indicates

   a. obsessional thoughts
   b. phobias
   c. delusional ideations
   d. compulsive behavior

   A. a
   B. a and b
   C. a and c
   D. a, c, and d   (4:65)

8. The major fundamental mechanism in hypochondriacal neurosis is

   A. repression
   B. regression
   C. rationalization
   D. conversion   (21:162–63)

9. A person with a phobia utilizes the defense mechanisms of

   A. repression, symbolization, and displacement
   B. repression, projection, and displacement
   C. symbolization and displacement
   D. repression, substitution, and displacement   (20:109)

10. Conversion reactions, hysterical type, are *not* usually

    A. diagnosed in women
    B. treated with electroshock therapy
    C. treated with psychotherapy
    D. life-threatening to the client   (10:274)

11. Psychological invalidism is another term for

    A. malingering
    B. neurasthenic neurosis
    C. hypochondriacal neurosis
    D. conversion reaction   (13:203)

12. Initially in a conversion reaction, hysterical type, it is common to find

    A. atrophy
    B. normal reflexes
    C. severe anxiety
    D. mild depression   (26:463)

13. The finding that anxiety constituted a major portion of the psychiatric casualties in World War II, in contrast to those of World War I, is best explained by the fact that

    A. anxiety is more characteristic of contempory society
    B. soldiers received more personal attention during World War II
    C. internists diagnosed anxiety as a cardiac disorder
    D. psychiatric illness held less of a stigma
    (6:III:216)

14. A repetitious symptom can be labeled obsessive or compulsive when it is

    A. not willingly accepted
    B. not willingly accepted and ego alien
    C. inconsistent as well as repetitious
    D. intrusive and bizarre   (6:III:216)

15. A basic psychodynamic explanation of obsessive behavior postulates that

    A. defiant rage overcomes guilty fear
    B. dependence overcomes independence
    C. guilty fear overcomes defiant rage
    D. independence overcomes dependence
    (6:III:198)

Directions: MATCH the following numbered items with the most appropriate lettered items.

The following are theories of anxiety. The choices are the theorists most associated with the theory.

Questions 16 to 20

E 16. The birth trauma is the prototype for anxiety
    (26:135)
C 17. Unconscious instinctual drives are the basis of anxiety   (26:135)
D 18. Anxiety as experienced as the anticipated disapproval or loss of love from one's significant others   (26:135–36)
B 19. Anxiety and hostility are centrally related
    (26:136)
A 20. Anxiety states are actually states of loneliness or fear of loneliness   (26:136)

A. Frieda Fromm-Reichmann
B. Karen Horney
C. Sigmund Freud
D. Harry Stack Sullivan
E. Otto Rank

Directions: For each of the following multiple choice questions, select the ONE most appropriate answer.

21. Which of the following parts of the body is most often involved in obsessive rituals?

    A. mouth
    B. anus
    C. extremities
    D. bladder   (6:III:202)

22. Examples of secondary gains from neurotic symptoms include

    a. control over important people
    b. enslaving a dominant spouse
    c. disguised gratification of the warded off wish
    d. temporary freedom from work demands

    A. a and d
    B. b, c, and d
    C. b and c
    D. a, b, and d   (6:III:20)

23. Hollingshead and Redlich suggest that upper class psychiatric patients tend to be

    A. obsessive or depressed
    B. anxious
    C. hypochondriacal or somatically expressive
    D. aggressive or resigned   (6:III:20)

24. In working with the patient who is diagnosed with a conversion reaction, the nurse shows understanding of the patient's needs if she

    A. focuses the patient's attention on his most prominent symptom
    B. evaluates his symptoms carefully
    C. does not express skepticism of the patient's oversimplified explanations

D. expects the patient to be astute in his observations of others   (18:353-55)

Questions 25 to 27

Miss Black is to be married in five days. She wakes up one morning and finds herself unable to speak. She seems calm about this although she has always been extroverted and likes to be in the limelight.

25. Miss Black is exhibiting

    a. conversion hysteria
    b. la belle indifference
    c. dissociation
    d. internal conflict

    A. a and b
    B. a, b, and c
    C. a, b, c, and d
    D. a, b, and d   (20:412–24)

26. Miss Black's behavior indicates the use of the defense mechanisms of

    a. repression
    b. symbolization
    c. undoing
    d. condensation

    A. a and b
    B. a and c
    C. b and c
    D. b and d   (20:418)

27. The primary gains from Miss Black's symptoms are

    a. the attention that she'll receive
    b. the solution of the internal conflict
    c. the postponement of the wedding
    d. the reduction of anxiety

    A. a, b, c, and d
    B. a and b
    C. a and c
    D. b and d   (20:418)

Questions 28 to 33

Cathy Thompson, a 35-year-old female, has been a patient in a psychiatric hospital for more than a year. She has a habit of washing her hands repeatedly for long periods of time.

28. The most basic purpose of ritualistic behavior such as Ms. Thompson's handwashing is to

    A. reduce the probability of infection
    B. occupy the mind with seemingly purposeful activity
    C. relieve one's anxiety
    D. manipulate one's environment   (20:425)

29. Which statement is generally true of a patient with ritualistic behavior?

    A. if the patient can be made to understand that the behavior is unreasonable, she will stop it
    B. the frequency of performance of the ritual is unrelated to the degree of anxiety
    C. the patient may be aware that the ritual is illogical, but she is helpless to stop it
    D. the patient is likely to be unaware that she is performing the ritual   (20:425)

30. One night the nurse interrupts Ms. Thompson's ritual and attempts to escort her to bed. Ms. Thompson slaps the nurse. The *most* probable reason for Ms. Thompson's response is

    A. she dislikes the nurse as a person
    B. she resents regulations such as bedtime hours
    C. ritualistic behavior is usually accompanied by acts of overt aggression
    D. because her ritual was not completed, she experienced excessive anxiety
                                           (20:426)

31. Later, Ms. Thompson approaches the nurse and says, "I'm sorry I slapped you. I don't know what made me do it." Which reply by the nurse would be *most* appropriate?

    A. "I've really forgotten all about it."
    B. "It's not pleasant to be slapped. Can we talk about how you felt?"
    C. "I'm glad you realize it and are sorry about this."
    D. "You really surprised me. I didn't expect it."   (26:172–73)

32. Ritualistic behavior is most commonly seen in the patient who is

    A. aggressive
    B. suspicious
    C. depressed
    D. compulsive   (20:425)

33. A physician is assigned as primary therapist to Ms. Thompson. The most appropriate role of the nurse would be to

    A. encourage her to explore the basis for her ritualistic behavior
    B. listen to her and communicate the details of her behavior
    C. suggest that she tell the therapist about her childhood
    D. explain to her why she should talk only to her therapist   (2:422)

34. The symptoms in a conversion reaction

    A. are under voluntary control
    B. control anxiety and relieve tension
    C. are the result of fantasies
    D. are a form of malingering   (26:463)

35. In implosive therapy, the phobic client is

    A. presented with graded intensities of the phobic threat
    B. instructed to interrupt the presentation of the phobic threat if anxiety occurs
    C. presented with massive exposure to the phobic object
    D. taught relaxation exercises   (6:III:130)

36. In neurotic depression, the client is apt to be *less* interested in activities

    A. in the morning
    B. in the early evening
    C. done in a group setting
    D. of a repetitive nature   (21:232)

37. Psychoneurotic patients who seek psychiatric treatment are usually from

    A. the higher socio-economic classes
    B. the middle socio-economic classes
    C. the lower socio-economic classes
    D. all socio-economic classes   (18:337)

38. Miss Samuels is a newly admitted client who has a phobia of elevators. The nurse who cares for Miss Samuels should understand that Miss Samuels

    A. may recognize her fear is irrational
    B. has repressed dependency needs
    C. probably has little insight
    D. is apt to be depressed   (20:408–09)

39. An obsessive compulsive neurosis is characterized by

    a. the expression of unconscious conflict through physical disturbances
    b. the presence of fixed, well-systematized delusions
    c. compelling, repetitive, and ritualistic patterns of thinking and behaving
    d. the absence of reality testing

    A. a and c
    B. a, c, and d
    C. c
    D. b and d   (20:425)

40. Mrs. Mason is experiencing an acute anxiety attack. Mrs. Lee, the nurse, is going to give her a mild sedative as prescribed. Mrs. Lee would indicate the *best* understanding of Mrs. Mason if she says

    A. "Mrs. Mason, the doctor ordered this for you."
    B. "Mrs. Mason, this should help you to feel more comfortable."
    C. "Mrs. Mason, this medication is to help you feel less anxious. Your anxiety is causing your symptoms."
    D. "Mrs. Mason, I know you feel nervous. This medicine will help you."   (2:156)

41. Which factor is likely to *increase* the nurse's *difficulty* in maintaining a professional role with a psychoneurotic patient?

    A. the patient's behavior is obviously pathological
    B. the patient is rarely communicative
    C. the patient reveals highly personalized information about himself

D. the patient attempts to form a social relationship (18:340)

Directions: MATCH the following numbered items with the most appropriate lettered items in relation to defense mechanisms in psychoneuroses.

Questions 42 to 46

42. Undoing (20:426)
43. Displacement (20:409)
44. Introjection (20:430–31)
45. Dissociation (20:410–11)
46. Conversion (20:406)

    A. Reactive depression
    B. Multiple personality
    C. Hysterical blindness
    D. Phobic reaction
    E. Obsessive-compulsive reactions

Directions: For each of the following multiple choice questions, select the ONE most appropriate answer.

47. The novel, *Dr. Jekyll and Mr. Hyde,* is a literary model of a

    A. dissociative syndrome
    B. paranoid reaction
    C. obsessive-compulsive reaction
    D. hysterical conversion (6:III:160)

48. Which of the following statements about a patient suffering from a conversion reaction is true?

    A. the symptom usually involves a function under control of the involuntary nervous system
    B. the conversion reaction is a symbolic expression of an inner conflict
    C. the anxiety arising out of the conflictive situation is primarily conscious
    D. the patient suffering from a conversion reaction is overtly anxious (26:462–64)

49. The most important characteristic of the nurse who is caring for a client with a severe anxiety attack is

    A. matter-of-factness
    B. calmness
    C. flexibility
    D. openness (2:156–57)

50. A patient who suffers from chronic anxiety states would usually benefit from

    A. frequent rest periods
    B. vacations
    C. purposeful activity
    D. "self-help" books (2:160)

51. An important aspect of nursing care of the hospitalized compulsive client is to

    A. increase his interpersonal interaction
    B. ignore the compulsive behavior
    C. utilize humor whenever possible
    D. allow the client to structure his activities (2:174–75)

52. Mr. Kelly has many physical complaints. He has had a complete physical examination and laboratory studies. No physical problems have been identified and his symptoms appear to be the result of anxiety. He requests that the nurse check his blood pressure several times a day. The nursing action that would be most appropriate is

    A. tell him that there is no physical problem and not to worry
    B. take his blood pressure and reassure him it is normal
    C. ask him to keep a record of his B/P readings
    D. listen to his complaints and encourage him to focus his interest on other topics or activities (26:468)

53. The phobic client controls his unacceptable feelings and impulses through

    A. symbolic and ritualistic activity
    B. dissociation and displacement to the environment
    C. repression and projection
    D. acting out behavior (4:73)

54. Which kind of neurotic symptoms are readily affected by suggestive procedures?

    A. phobias
    B. hysterical reaction
    C. anxiety states
    D. obsessive-compulsive reactions   (2:181)

Directions: MATCH the number of the descriptive item with the letter of the appropriate phobia.

Questions 55 to 64

55. Fear of heights   (7:24)
56. Fear of darkness   (7:1393)
57. Fear of dirt and germs   (7:1003)
58. Fear of closed spaces   (7:320)
59. Fear of water   (7:120, 720)
60. Fear of stating that which is not absolutely
    correct   (7:1003)
61. Fear of open places   (7:47)
62. Fear of fire   (7:1293)
63. Fear of spiders   (7:121)
64. Fear of being alone   (7:972)

    A. Aquaphobia
    B. Pyrophobia
    C. Acrophobia
    D. Agoraphobia
    E. Scotophobia
    F. Mythophobia
    G. Claustrophobia
    H. Mysophobia
    I. Monophobia
    J. Arachnephobia

Directions: For each of the following multiple choice questions, select the ONE most appropriate answer.

65. Which of the following statements describe the Ganser syndrome?

    a. it is a rare type of hysterical dissociative reaction
    b. it is a type of malingered illness
    c. it occurs in prisoners awaiting trial
    d. it occurs in enlisted military men

    A. a and c
    B. b and d
    C. a and d
    D. b and c   (2:178–79)

66. Obsessive patients are characterized by the fact that there is

    A. an urge to carry out the obsessive thought
    B. a dread that the obsession will occur
    C. a combination of urgency to enact and dread of the obsessive thought
    D. an underlying thought disorder   (2:167)

67. Which of the following are seen in all psychoneurotic sub-types *except* the conversion reaction?

    A. repression
    B. anxiety
    C. negativism
    D. rationalization   (18:340–52)

68. The type of psychoneurosis that one develops is related to

    a. social factors
    b. economic factors
    c. cultural factors
    d. genetic factors

    A. a and b
    B. b and d
    C. a, c, and d
    D. a, b and c   (18:337)

69. Psychoneurotic symptoms are usually observed as

    A. single neurotic reactions
    B. the only psychological pathology
    C. admixtures of neurotic reactions
    D. reactions to extreme external stress
                                           (18:337)

Questions 70 to 74

Mr. Brown is a 45-year-old patient with a diagnosis of obsessive-compulsive neurosis. His ritualistic behavior consists of handwashing. He also has a phobia of being surrounded by people.

70. Miss Smith, a new nurse, introduces herself to Mr. Brown and asks his name. He responds, "I am an obsessive-compulsive neu-

rotic. I have had psychoanalysis for 20 years. What do you think you can do for me?" The nursing response that would be most helpful is

A. "Who was your analyst, Mr. Brown?"
B. "You seem to feel hopeless, Mr. Brown."
C. "I need to know you better, Mr. Brown."
D. "Can we talk about that, Mr. Brown"?
(10:92)

71. Mr. Brown is getting on the elevator for occupational therapy. Suddenly he says to the nurse, "I need to go wash my hands." The most therapeutic action would be to

A. tell Mr. Brown he can wash his hands when he gets to occupational therapy
B. tell Mr. Brown that you understand how he feels and that you'll stay with him
C. tell Mr. Brown that you will take him back to the unit
D. ask Mr. Brown why he needs to wash his hands (9:84–5)

72. The nurse should expect that Mr. Brown will experience less anxiety if he is

A. allowed to return to the unit and wash his hands
B. asked to express why he needs to wash his hands
C. allowed to make as many decisions as possible for his own care
D. able to delay washing his hands until he gets to O.T. (9:86)

73. The handwashing ritual demonstrates the use of the defense mechanism of

A. denial
B. suppression
C. undoing
D. projection (20:427)

74. An obsession is best described as

A. a persistent, unwanted thought
B. an automatic thought
C. a recurrent thought
D. a fixed idea (20:108)

75. The most frequent neurotic problem in outpatient psychiatric work is

A. severe phobias
B. obsessive-compulsive patterns
C. anxiety states
D. reactive depressions (2:161)

76. A severely phobic patient who suppresses all angry feelings needs an attitude of

A. active friendliness
B. passive friendliness
C. permissiveness
D. pleasant firmness (2:390–91)

77. Mrs. Bleeker is a 56-year-old housewife. She has a history of many somatic complaints with no physical origin. She bitterly complains that some of the staff neglect her. Miss Snow, a nurse, tries to give her special attention and is annoyed with her coworkers. The best action on the part of Miss Snow would be to

A. observe if other staff neglect Mrs. Bleeker
B. continue to give Mrs. Bleeker special attention
C. chart Mrs. Bleeker's remarks
D. ask that Mrs. Bleeker's care be the topic of the next ward conference
(2:399)

Questions 78 to 80

Mrs. Paula Kraft is a 30-year-old client, married and the mother of two children. One morning she is playing a game with a group in which she is well accepted. She begins to perspire profusely, tremble, and to breathe with apparent difficulty. She has an intense, worried expression on her face. She says, "I don't know what it is, but something dreadful is happening to me."

78. Which of the following phrases best describe what Mrs. Kraft is experiencing?

A. a false perception
B. separation anxiety
C. severe anxiety
D. conversion hysteria (6:III:94–5)

79. Which one of the following comments by the nurse would be most helpful?

   A. "Relax, Mrs. Kraft. Nothing is going to happen."
   B. "I'll get you some medicine to quiet your nerves."
   C. "Mrs. Kraft, I think it's best if you go to your room and rest."
   D. "I'll stay here with you until you feel calmer." (18:349)

80. Mrs. Kraft tells the nurse that tomorrow is her daughter's birthday. She hopes that her daughter will like her gift. Which one of the following factors was probably primarily responsible for precipitating this episode?

   A. a "stirring up" of a forgotten painful experience
   B. a feeling of guilt about being away from home for her daughter's birthday
   C. a concern that her daughter will not like her birthday gift
   D. a desire to secure more attention for herself (26:459)

81. Amnesia is self-deception through
   A. disguise
   B. dissociation
   C. reaction-formation
   D. regression (10:409)

82. Which of the following is *not* characteristic of a conversion reaction?

   A. la belle indifference
   B. involvement of the autonomic nervous system
   C. the symbolic nature of the symptom
   D. relief of anxiety (20:412)

83. All of the following statements about phobias are ture *except*

   A. the phobic reaction per se is diagnosed infrequently
   B. phobics are usually concerned with the avoidance of aggression
   C. the phobic uses avoidance as a primary means of resolving problems

   D. phobias are twice as common among men as among women (20:408–09)

B. Personality Disorders

Directions: For each of the following multiple choice questions, select the ONE most appropriate answer.

Questions 84 to 89

Doris Green, an attractive 24-year-old young woman, is admitted to a psychiatric unit with the diagnosis of antisocial personality disturbance.

84. The essential defect in the character structure of the person with an antisocial personality rests in

   A. failure to express basic id impulses
   B. failure to develop a socialized superego and ego ideals
   C. an early symbiotic relationship with the mothering one
   D. lack of adequate ego boundaries (20:496)

85. Which type of behavior would be most typical for this patient?

   A. withdrawing from social activities
   B. following ward routine with mechanical obedience
   C. utilizing rituals to allay anxiety
   D. seeking special privileges (20:496)

86. Which of the following factors are frequently found in the developmental history of the antisocial personality?

   A. born out of wedlock
   B. history of foster homes or orphanages
   C. open rebellion against a dominating parent
   D. all of the above (20:496)

87. Which combination of responses would a nurse be likely to observe in Doris?

   A. unsociable, seclusive, and autistic behavior

B. amoral, unreliable, and unpredictable behavior

C. negativistic, suspicious, and eccentric behavior

D. stereotyped, silly, and bizarre behavior
(20:496–98)

88. Which of the following measures should receive the greatest emphasis for a patient with an antisocial personality?

A. assisting the patient to participate in recreational activities

B. offering the patient the opportunity to make simple choices

C. enlisting the aid of an occupational therapist to provide manual activities for the patient

D. setting and enforcing reasonable limits for the patient's conduct on the ward
(20:500–01)

89. When Doris' parents visit, they ask the nurse about Doris' chances of getting well. Which reply by the nurse would be most helpful to the parents?

A. "Unfortunately, patients like your daughter rarely get well, but with proper attention, they are able to adjust satisfactorily."

B. "I've seen patients like your daughter before and they usually respond well to treatment; however, it would be better for you to ask her doctor."

C. "We are all very concerned with helping Doris. If you wish, I'll be glad to make an appointment for you to see her doctor."

D. "I'm not permitted to say anything. You will have to see her doctor for such information."
(20:500)

90. Which of the following percentages account for the number of persons who are "skid row" type alcoholics?

A. 25%
B. 75%
C. 30%
D. 5%
(13:334)

91. Which of the following persons is most likely to be alcoholic?

A. a high school graduate
B. a white-collar worker
C. a lawyer
D. an umemployed grammar school graduate
(13:334-36)

92. Bulimia is another term for

A. polyphagia
B. anorexia nervosa
C. dysphagia
D. pica
(4:16)

93. The excessive use of alcohol to help a person function in a situation that he finds difficult can be referred to as

A. social alcoholism
B. neurotic alcoholism
C. psychotic alcoholism
D. sporadic drinking
(10:360)

94. Denial of the problem is typically the first phase of the reaction of families of clients with the diagnosis of

A. alcoholism
B. sociopathic personality
C. conversion hysteria
D. schizophrenia
(27:II:173)

95. Which of the following blood alcohol percentages indicates the least amount of alcohol that causes intoxication in a 150 pound person?

A. 0.05 to 0.10%
B. 0.10 to 0.20%
C. 0.20 to 0.30%
D. 0.30 to 0.40%
(13:332)

96. In caring for the client with delirium tremens, all of the following measures are appropriate except

A. the room should be well lighted
B. the environment should be non-stimulating
C. bed rails and/or restraints should be utilized
D. procedures should be kept to a minimum
(2:311)

97. In America, alcoholism is estimated to have an impact on the families of

    A. 2 million persons
    B. 10 million persons
    C. 20 million persons
    D. 25 million persons   (10:358)

98. Alcoholics and narcotic addicts differ in which of the following areas?

    a. release of sexual drives
    b. release of aggressive drives
    c. work performance
    d. criminality of the dependence

    A. a and b
    B. c and d
    C. a and c
    D. b, c, and d   (18:398–99)

99. Mrs. Smith is described as a demanding patient. She refuses to go to occupational therapy. Miss Johnson is the nurse assigned to care for Mrs. Smith for the day. Which of the following actions is most appropriate initially?

    A. to chart Mrs. Smith's behavior
    B. to explain the purpose of occupational therapy
    C. to tell Mrs. Smith she is expected to go to occupational therapy
    D. to provide Mrs. Smith with activities to do on the unit   (13:264)

100. Which of the following statements about alcohol is true?

    A. alcohol is useful in assisting one to keep warm in a cold climate
    B. beer has insufficient alcohol to produce intoxication
    C. alcohol is a stimulant
    D. alcohol in moderate amounts can aid digestion   (13:332)

101. Which of the following characteristics is common to all alcoholics?

    a. narcissism
    b. latent homosexuality

    c. strong oral drives
    d. excessive alcohol intake

    A. a and d
    B. c and d
    C. a, c, and d
    D. d only   (13:331)

102. Features of sexual behavior that are considered deviant in adults

    A. never occur in normal persons
    B. seldom occur in normal children
    C. frequently occur in normal children
    D. never occur in normal children (26:480)

103. Another term for a "peeping Tom" is

    A. an exhibitionist
    B. a voyeur
    C. a fetishist
    D. a pedophil   (4:90)

Questions 104 to 106

Miss Rivers, an attractive 25-year-old woman, is admitted to a psychiatric unit and diagnosed as having an antisocial personality.

104. One would expect Miss Rivers to

    A. follow the rules of the unit
    B. observe the power structure of the unit
    C. avoid socializing with the other patients
    D. pretend to desire hospitalization
                                (10:224)

105. Miss Rivers is probably adept at

    A. controlling her own feelings
    B. sizing up others
    C. empathizing with fellow patients
    D. being a "model" patient   (6:III:258)

106. One day, Miss Rivers impulsively attacks another patient whom she feels has been intruding on her privacy for some time. Which action by the nurse is appropriate?

    A. keep Miss Rivers away from other patients

B. disregard this incident, but suggest to Miss Rivers that she may be disciplined if it occurs again

C. disregard the incident since it is important that Miss Rivers act out her unconscious needs

D. intervene actively to stop the fight and discuss the incident with Miss Rivers

(18:385)

Questions 107 to 110

Mr. Flynn has been drinking periodically for 15 years. He entered the hospital after he was no longer able to work or function in any way without the aid of a "couple of shots." He is contrite and apologetic and states frequently, "I'll never drink again." Mrs. Flynn has left her husband on numerous occasions but always returns when he promises to stop drinking as she feels he couldn't manage without her.

107. The nursing approach to Mr. Flynn should take into consideration that

A. he has a strong need for punishment and this need should be met by the staff

B. he has a tendency to lie about giving up alcohol and these lies should be pointed out to him by the staff

C. he has a severe loss of self-esteem and therefore his ego should be strengthened whenever possible

D. from now on he will have to limit his drinking to social gatherings if he is really sincere about controlling his alcoholism (26:402)

108. Alcohol serves all of the following purposes for the alcoholic *except* that it

A. reduces dependency needs
B. satisfies oral needs
C. decreases superego controls
D. lessens control of fantasies (26:402)

109. The nursing measure that would be most helpful to Mr. Flynn during periods of delirium tremens would include

A. asking the physician for an order for Thorazine 100 mg I.M.

B. assuring the patient that he has nothing to worry about because his illusions are not real

C. minimizing external stimuli to lessen frightening illusions

D. using the experience to point out to him the dangers of over-indulgence

(26:407–08)

110. The nurse refers Mrs. Flynn to Alanon. Alanon endeavors to help members to

A. learn about the effects of their relationship with the alcoholic partner

B. get psychiatric treatment

C. become financially independent of their spouses

D. understand their alcoholic spouses

(26:409)

Directions: MATCH the following numbered items with the most appropriate lettered items.

Questions 111 to 117

111. inept, exercise poor judgement, lack stamina
(26:474)

112. F aloof, fearful, eccentric, introverted
(26:475)

A 113. D enthusiastic, friendly, competitive
(26:475)

114. B suspicious, jealous, stubborn, envious
(26:475)

C 115. A excitable, sulky, irritable, unpredictable
(26:476)

D 116. helpless, indecisive, procrastinating, resentful
(26:476–77)

117. E rigid, meticulous, perfectionistic, conforming
(26:477)

A. Cyclothymic personality
B. Paranoid personality
C. Emotionally unstable personality
D. Passive-aggressive personality
E. Compulsive personality
F. Schizoid personality
G. Inadequate personality

Directions: For each of the following multiple choice questions, select the ONE most appropriate answer.

118. Which of the following factors influence the prognosis in drug addiction?

    A. the client's age
    B. the educational level of the client
    C. the employment record of the client
    D. all of the above   (30:155)

119. Possible etiological factors in the development of homosexuality in a male include

    a. identification with the mother
    b. role reversal of the parents
    c. coed boarding school during adolescence
    d. imprisonment during adolescence

    A. a and b
    B. b and c
    C. b, c, and d
    D. a, b, and d   (18:117)

120. Which of the following approaches to group work is characteristic of Alcoholics Anonymous?

    A. spontaneity approach
    B. client-centered approach
    C. repressive inspirational approach
    D. direct approach   (27:I:249)

121. Which factors support and perpetuate addictive disorders?

    a. The fear of the withdrawal phenomena
    b. the fear of survival in the "straight world"
    c. the attraction to the comfort of the addiction
    d. The ritualism of the addiction

    A. a, b, and c
    B. b and c
    C. a and d
    D. a, b, c, and d   (30:150)

122. The successful treatment of the client with an antisocial reaction disorder (sociopath) probably always requires that

    A. the client be in an institution
    B. the staff be well trained and devoted
    C. there be job training
    D. there be group and individual therapy
                (6:III:265)

123. Which of the following psychotherapists are noted for their writings about antisocial behavior?

    a. H. Cleckley
    b. T. Capote
    c. A. Aichhorn
    d. T. Szasz

    A. a and b
    B. a and c
    C. a, b, and c
    D. a, b, c, and d   (6:III:258:260)

124. An important reason for the team approach in the treatment of the alcoholic is that it permits

    A. more alcoholics to be treated as it is economical
    B. the staff to share the supervision of clients who tend to be manipulative
    C. the clients to interact with a variety of professionals
    D. the hostility of the alcoholic to be shared   (18:411–12)

125. Bill is a 22-year-old homosexual client who has been admitted to the hospital because of a suicidal attempt. It is probable that

    A. there is a relationship between the homosexuality and the suicide attempt
    B. Bill has a seductive rejecting mother
    C. Bill has suffered a loss of love
    D. his homosexual relationships have been promiscuous   (20:98)

126. Which of the following characteristics describe Synanon, an agency dedicated to the treatment of drug addiction?

a. addicts volunteer for treatment
b. addicts are withdrawn without the support of drugs
c. addicts are withdrawn from their habit without the supervision of a physician
d. it is an organization of former addicts

A. a and b
B. b and c
C. a and d
D. a, b, c, and d   (18:403)

127. In which way does a synanon differ from other forms of group therapy?

A. they are generally held three times a week
B. they are composed of 12 to 15 people
C. they are led by older and more experienced members
D. the membership of a synanon is different at each session   (18:408)

128. What is the greatest drawback to the successful treatment of the alcoholic?

A. the lack of theory about alcoholism
B. the lack of motivation on the part of the alcoholic
C. the lack of comprehensive preparation for practice in nursing schools
D. the antipathy and lack of understanding of the therapist   (18:411)

129. The U.S. Public Health Service aids in the treatment of narcotic addiction through

A. two federal hospitals
B. Synanon and Narcotics Anonymous
C. a federal prison system
D. a training program for medical doctors
                                     (18:400)

130. Fatalities among narcotic addicts are usually the result of

A. unsupervised withdrawal from the drug
B. contaminated needles and syringes
C. overdosage of the drug
D. accidentally repeating the drug after a brief interval   (20:514)

131. Which three variables are essential in becoming addicted to drugs?

a. a psychologically maladjusted individual
b. a source of supply
c. a psychological crisis
d. an available drug

A. a, b, and c
B. b, c, and d
C. a, b, and c
D. a, c, and d   (18:399)

132. The person predisposed to narcotic addiction most often becomes addicted by being

A. coaxed into use by a "pusher"
B. introduced to drugs by his associates
C. exposed to drugs in a medical situation
D. purposeful in his pursuit of sources of drugs   (18:399)

133. Alcohol addiction has withdrawal symptoms of

a. tremors, excessive perspiration, anorexia
b. hallucinations, restlessness
c. convulsions
d. nausea and vomiting

A. a and b
B. c and d
C. a, c, and d
D. a, b, c, and d   (18:387)

Questions 134 to 135

Mr. Jones is talking to Miss Brown the nurse. He states, "When I don't get my way, I do something about it. I show them who's boss. No one tells me what to do."

134. This is an example of

A. lack of impulse control
B. intimidating behavior
C. acting out behavior
D. lack of super-ego controls   (10:224)

135. Miss Brown's best initial response would be

    A. "Can you tell me more about how you feel?"
    B. "Are you trying to frighten me?"
    C. "I'm not telling you what to do."
    D. "Sounds like you have trouble with authority." (10:225)

136. A man who becomes sexually aroused only when he has contact with silk material is exhibiting

    A. fellatio
    B. transvestism
    C. fetishism
    D. erotomania (20:505)

137. Which factors are characteristic of personality disorders?

    a. faulty superego formation
    b. somatic symptoms predominate
    c. pathology is directed toward others
    d. pathology is expressed by the behavior

    A. a and b
    B. b, c, and d
    C. a, c, and d
    D. c and d (18:366)

138. Joseph Kelly has been admitted to the hospital following an arrest for stealing a car while under the influence of cocaine. He has been arrested before but has been paroled quickly for good behavior. He is a high school drop-out although his grades were above average. He has been diagnosed as a dissocial reaction. The nurse might expect that

    A. Joseph's superego controls are impaired
    B. Joseph is unable to sustain an intimate relationship
    C. Joseph does not consciously experience guilt and anxiety
    D. Joseph's family's values are different from society's in general (21:316)

139. Which environmental factor is likely to be most distressing to a patient with delirium tremens?

    A. presence of people
    B. shadows
    C. wood odors
    D. noise (26:407)

140. Which immediate nursing measure is most appropriate in relieving severe pain in the lower extremities of the patient with delirium tremens?

    A. use of a bed cradle to relieve the lower extremities of the weight of the bed clothing
    B. massage the legs with warm oil
    C. elevate the legs on pillows
    D. apply ice bags over the course of the major nerves of the lower extremities (20:214)

141. Which additional measure is important in caring for the client's acute neuropathy?

    A. support his feet in dorsiflexion
    B. encourage him to exercise his legs in bicycling motions
    C. be certain that his lower extremities are in external rotation while he is recumbent
    D. place one hand under the mid-thigh and the other under the mid-calf in moving his lower extremities. (20:214)

142. Which activity is within the stated functions of Alcoholics Anonymous?

    A. using psychotherapy to help persons with alcoholism gain insight into the causes of their problems
    B. providing legal counseling for persons with alcoholism who get into legal difficulties
    C. financing therapeutic programs to assist persons with alcoholism
    D. providing supportive relationships for persons with alcoholism (21:326)

143. Which measure is especially important in the care of a patient with Korsakoff's psychosis?

    A. reminding him when scheduled activities are about to begin
    B. urging him to drink low caloric fluids

C. planning a nonstimulating environment
D. enrolling him in the gymnastic program
(20:214)

144. Which of the following measures should receive the greatest emphasis in the nursing care plan for a patient with an antisocial personality?

A. assisting the patient to participate in recreational activities
B. offering the patient opportunities in recreational activities
C. enlisting the aid of the occupational therapist in providing manual activities
D. setting and enforcing reasonable limits for the patient's conduct on the ward
(10:226)

145. John Petrie, 25 years of age, is a heroin addict who is admitted to a psychiatric hospital. Which sign is most indicative that he is using a drug such as heroin?

A. choreiform movements
B. excessive salivation
C. frequent coughing
D. pinpoint pupils
(10:368)

146. Opiate addiction is more common among

A. ghetto-dwellers and minority groups
B. middle class teenagers
C. upper class teenagers
D. college students
(10:367)

147. In planning care for the manipulative patient, it is important to

a. identify and acknowledge one's own uncomfortable feelings
b. understand the meaning of the behavior
c. assess how the patient understands what he does
d. validate the dynamics of the behavior with all the staff

A. a and b
B. a, b, and d
C. a, b, and c
D. a, b, c, and d
(10:225)

148. Miss Jones, a 17-year-old patient with a personality disorder, is observed by the nurse

banging her hand against the wall. The most appropriate nursing response would be

A. "Miss Jones, can we talk together about what is upsetting you?"
B. "Miss Jones, unless you stop, you'll have to have medication."
C. "Why are you banging your hand, Miss Jones?"
D. "Miss Jones, come and help me get some supplies."
(10:225)

149. Which of the following drugs produces no appreciable damage to bodily tissue even in the case of severe habituation?

a. alcohol
b. morphine
c. L.S.D.
d. marihuana

A. a and d
B. b and d
C. a and c
D. c and d
(2:324; 21:329)

150. One would expect the chronic user of amphetamines to be

A. energetic
B. underweight
C. overweight
D. depressed
(2:323)

151. The chronic user of amphetamines may develop psychotic symptoms. These are typically in the form of

A. depressive states
B. manic states
C. paranoid states
D. confused states
(2:323)

152. Which of the following statements about drug abuse is *in*correct?

A. addicts may fake physical symptoms in order to receive medications
B. social pressure is frequently a factor in abuse of drugs
C. health professionals have a low rate of incidence of drug abuse
D. withdrawal from morphine is not "life threatening"
(13:352)

153. Which of the following statements about alcoholism as an addictive reaction is *in*accurate?

    A. it is uncertain if a true physical addiction occurs with the chronic use of alcohol
    B. there is both psychological and physiological dependence on alcohol
    C. physical tolerance for alcohol is a typical feature
    D. death can occur from an "overdose" of alcohol (21:329)

154. If the nurse is to work comfortably as well as effectively with alcoholic patients, first she may need a chance to

    A. seek further clinical preparation
    B. examine her own feelings and reactions to alcoholic patients
    C. function well in crisis situations
    D. understand the community as well as the hosptial (21:412)

155. The medical profession, through the American Medical Association, first officially recognized alcoholism as an illness in

    A. 1944
    B. 1956
    C. 1918
    D. 1900 (18:386)

156. Alcoholism was first recognized as an illness, social problem, and social responsibility in the United States in

    A. 1952
    B. 1961
    C. 1944
    D. 1968 (26:401)

157. The most important aspects of the management of the patient with delirium tremens is to make certain the patient is

    a. receiving fluids
    b. undergoing electrolyte studies
    c. receiving paraldehyde
    d. physically restrained

    A. a only
    B. b only
    C. a and b
    D. c and d (6:III:381)

158. Delirium tremens is fatal in about

    A. 20% of untreated cases
    B. 10% of untreated cases
    C. 15% of untreated cases
    D. 5% of untreated cases (6:III:381)

159. Which of the following statements most accurately describes the progression of alcoholism?

    A. alcohol will eventually dominate one's life and cause social and physical deterioration
    B. there are a number of alternative courses for alcoholism to take including spontaneous recovery
    C. treatment is necessary to avoid becoming a skid row derelict
    D. the steady state drinker will remain in this pattern and not become a fluctuating drinker (6:III:379–80)

160. Which factors are *not* typical in the history of the client with antisocial behavior?

    a. college graduate
    b. married for ten years
    c. raised in a foster home
    d. good intelligence

    A. a and b
    B. a and c
    C. b and d
    D. c and d (6:III:258–61)

161. Which drinking practices indicate an understanding of the idea of responsible drinking?

    a. drinking small amounts, well-diluted and taken in combination with food
    b. finding congenial and relaxed settings
    c. avoiding drinking to relieve tension
    d. avoiding situations in which drinking is equated with manliness

A.   a and b
B.   b and c
C.   c and d
D.   a, b, c, and d   (6:III:386)

162.   The clinical course of narcotic addiction includes

A.   serious impairment of mind and body
B.   no evidence of mental deterioration
C.   pathology directly related to the opiate
D.   impairment of the mind   (6:III:397)

163.   Symptoms of withdrawal from heroin include

a.   lacrimation, yawning, sneezing
b.   shivering and neuromuscular twitching
c.   elevated blood pressure
d.   severe vomiting and diarrhea

A.   a and b
B.   a, b, and d
C.   c and d
D.   a, b, c, and d   (6:III:396)

164.   In caring for the client who is dependent upon amphetamines, the nurse would expect adverse effects consisting of

A.   withdrawal symptoms of loss of interest and hypochondriasis
B.   ideas of reference and paranoid ideas of a persecuting nature
C.   delirium and stupor
D.   bewilderment, incoherence, and poorly organized delusions   (6:III:424)

165.   Which of the following are psychotomimetic agents?

A.   LSD-25, mescaline, naloxone
B.   marihuana, LSD-25, psilocybin
C.   mescaline, naloxone, cyclazocine
D.   psilocybin, cocaine, mescaline
          (6:III:410–11)

166.   Psychological changes that occur in the alcoholic person include

a.   planning daily events around drinking
b.   rationalizing about drinking behavior
c.   having feelings of disgust
d.   being persistently remorseful

A.   a and c
B.   b, c, and d
C.   a and b
D.   a, b, c, and d   (6:III:378)

167.   All of these groups of symptoms may occur in the withdrawal of heroin. Which group is likely to occur *first*?

A.   cramps in visceral muscles, increase in leukocytes, disorientation
B.   restlessness, lacrimation, yawning, sneezing
C.   vomiting, diarrhea, general prostration
D.   dilated pupils, irregular pulse, exhaustion   (10:368)

168.   Which of the following statements about pedophilics are true?

a.   they are male
b.   they are female
c.   sexual preference is for girls under age 16
d.   sexual preference is for boys under age 16

A.   a and c
B.   b and d
C.   a, c, and d
D.   a, b, c, and d   (12:205)

169.   Which of the following statements about transvestites is/are true?

a.   all transvestites are men
b.   most transvestites are heterosexual
c.   many transvestites are married
d.   many transvestites have children

A.   a only
B.   a and b
C.   c and d
D.   a, b, c, and d   (12:214)

170. When the putting on of clothes of the opposite sex produces unquestioned genital excitement which often leads to masturbation and orgasm, the condition is called

   A. homosexuality
   B. transexualism
   C. transvestism
   D. fetishism (12:214)

171. Findings from the Wolfendon Report in England on homosexuality and prostitution include all *except*

   A. most homosexual behavior is not forced on either partner
   B. most homosexuals are not sexually interested in children or adolescents
   C. homosexual activity in adulthood is usually a result of homosexual seduction in childhood
   D. homosexuals often get into trouble with the law (12:211)

172. Miss Anthony, the attractive 17-year-old daughter of a prominent citizen, is admitted to a psychiatric hospital for treatment of drug addiction. Miss Anthony is addicted to heroin. Which one of these statements expresses what is probably the most serious ill effect of drug addiction on the adolescent?

   A. it produces irreversible brain damage
   B. it causes the individual to live in a world of delusions
   C. it arrests development at a dependent stage
   D. it deprives the individual of a sense of accomplishment (20:514–19)

C. Psychosomatic Disorders

Directions: For each of the following multiple choice questions, select the ONE most appropriate answer.

173. Mr. Davitz, a 56-year-old accountant, has recently been asked to retire. Two weeks prior to the nurse's interview, Mr. Davitz developed gastric bleeding. His stress response is *most* closely related to

   A. threat of bodily injury
   B. loss of something highly valued
   C. frustration of sexual drives
   D. fear of financial reverses (25:183)

174. The nurse's intervention with Mr. Davitz would include

   a. helping him to identify interpersonal resources
   b. helping him to regain employment
   c. supporting his decision-making ability
   d. helping him to move to a less expensive neighborhood

   A. a only
   B. b only
   C. a and c
   D. b and d (1:84–8)

175. Asthma is considered a psychophysiological disease because

   A. persons affected have the same psychological makeup
   B. pollution always activates the General Adaptation Syndrome
   C. emotional factors influence the onset and occurence of physiological changes
   D. the illness is mental and emotional (20:473)

176. Pronounced dependency longings including a denial of and reaction-formation against these longings characterize to a large degree, the patient who is suffering from

   A. ulcerative colitis
   B. peptic ulcer
   C. essential hypertension
   D. rheumatoid arthritis (20:459)

177. Pseudocyesis strongly indicates a basic conflict over

   A. autonomy
   B. dependency
   C. aggressive impulses
   D. childbearing (20:482)

178. Psychophysiologic disorders are characterized by

    a. physical symptoms
    b. emotional conflict
    c. primary gains
    d. structural changes

    A. a and b
    B. a, b, and d
    C. b and d
    D. a and d   (21:347)

179. One of the major psychodynamic explanations for understanding a person with asthma is

    A. the client is directly expressing his anger
    B. the client is unconsciously wishing to die
    C. the client is symbolically asking for attention from a mothering figure
    D. the client is symbolically suffering from a physiological condition   (13:200)

180. Mr. Greene is 10 days postoperative for a colon resection and has a temporary colostomy. He refuses to look at the stoma and defers offers of teaching, stating, "My wife will care for it at home." His behavior most likely indicates

    a. the use of the defense mechanism of denial
    b. excessive dependency on his wife as a sick role behavior
    c. an adequate way of coping with a temporary change
    d. a possible reflection of his personality prior to illness

    A. b only
    B. b and d
    C. a, c, and d
    D. a, b, and d   (20:83)

181. Psychotic symptoms can occur in

    a. cardiac diseases
       liver disorders
    c. kidney disorders
    d. endocrine disorders

    A. a, d, and c
    B. a and b
    C. c and d
    D. a, b, c, and d   (10:280–81)

182. The theory that the common cold is a symptom of depression views the common cold as a

    A. conversion reaction
    B. psychophysiologic disorder
    C. hypochondriacal reaction
    D. normal form of mourning   (10:268)

183. Which of the following characteristics is *not* typical of patients with peptic ulcers?

    A. treatment may be provided by various medical specialists
    B. surgery may be necessary in the treatment
    C. an "ulcer type" of personality is present
    D. ulcers occur most frequently in male adults   (21:355–56)

184. A young woman was unable to express her grief at the time of her mother's death. Recently every time her boyfriend sent her flowers, she had an asthmatic attack. In therapy, she recalls that there were similar flowers in her mother's coffin. This is an example of a

    A. conversion reaction
    B. reactive depression
    C. psychophysiologic disorder
    D. dissociative reaction   (13:194)

Questions 185 to 187

Mr. Gleason, a married man with three children, has been on the medical ward for five days with the diagnosis of hypertension. He seems tense but denies he is really sick. While talking with Mr. Gleason, Mr. Clark, the nurse, learns that Mr. Gleason feels that his hypertension is caused by his children's constant fighting. Mr. Clark notes that when Mr. Gleason's wife and children come in, the children begin to argue.

185. The best initial action for Mr. Clark to take, would be to

    A. ask the children to stop the arguing as their father is ill
    B. ask the children to leave the room
    C. ask the children if they would like to go to the coffee shop
    D. ask Mr. Gleason if this behavior is upsetting to him   (10:265–66)

186. Mr. Clark might *best* prevent future episodes of this behavior by

    A. telling Mrs. Gleason to leave the children at home
    B. talking with the children after the visit and allowing them to discuss their feelings about the hospitalization
    C. talking with the children after the visit about their role in their father's illness
    D. asking Mrs. Gleason to be more active in disciplining the children   (10:265)

187. After the visit, Mr. Gleason says to Mr. Clark, "See what I mean, those kids of mine are always at one another. My wife just says that all kids act this way." Mr. Clark would be most helpful if he responded by saying

    A. "Perhaps your wife should see our social worker."
    B. "You are angry with your wife's attitude."
    C. "Don't be embarrassed. I've seen kids argue before."
    D. "You find that their arguing upsets you."   (10:265)

Questions 188 to 189

Mr. Gallagher has been admitted to the hospital for a G.I. series. He is suspected of having a peptic ulcer. Mr. Gallagher, a stock broker, is married and the father of three children.

188. The nurse should recognize that Mr. Gallagher's disorder is a psychophysiologic one which means that his ulcer represents

    A. repressed aggressive strivings
    B. unfulfilled dependency strivings

    C. a direct symbolic expression of conflict
    D. a reaction to stress   (20:449–59)

189. Mr. Gallagher undergoes a gastrectomy. He is cooperative and cheerful. It seems important to him that he appear "in control" and stalwart. He rarely complains of pain. When Mrs. Murphy, the nurse, comes into his room, he remarks, "My doctor will be in today. He said that I may go home tomorrow. I was worried that it might be too soon, but he should know his business. He's top-notch in the field, so it's best that I do what he says. That's what I'm paying for." Mrs. Murphy's best initial response would be

    A. "Yes, Dr. Jones is the best. He's quite respected."
    B. "You're afraid that you're too weak to go home."
    C. "Dr. Jones usually discharges his patients at this point."
    D. "You're wondering if Dr. Jones will decide if it's safe for you to go home tomorrow."   (9:132–33)

190. Characteristics of anorexia nervosa include

    a. restless activity
    b. amenorrhea and constipation
    c. reduction in intake
    d. weight loss

    A. a, b, and c
    B. a and d
    C. b and c
    D. a, b, c, and d   (20:465)

191. In caring for the client with anorexia nervosa, the problem of intake is a priority one. The nurse should intervene initially by

    A. force-feeding the client
    B. allowing the client to be alone at meal-times
    C. sitting with the client at meal-time
    D. spoon feeding the client   (13:202)

Questions 192 to 195

Mr. Smith is a mild-mannered, easy-going man with essential hypertension.

192. Which of the following is most apt to describe Mr. Smith?

   A. Mr. Smith suppresses his rage and utilizes the defense mechanism of reaction formation
   B. Mr. Smith suffers from arteriosclerosis
   C. Mr. Smith's pent-up rage is directly expressed via elevated blood pressure
   D. Mr. Smith is easy-going because his high blood pressure does not trouble him   (20:455–56)

193. Which of the following statements about essential hypertension are true?

   a. emotions seem to play a significant role in the production of the condition
   b. there is considerable evidence to suggest a hereditary element in this condition
   c. many hypertensives are neurotic with strong competitive drives
   d. the basic emotional conflict has usually originated in stress situations of early childhood

   A. a and b
   B. a and c
   C. a, c, and d
   D. a, b, c, and d   (20:455–56;21:345–46)

194. A mental mechanism commonly used by hypertensive patients such as Mr. Smith is

   A. dissociation
   B. denial
   C. sublimation
   D. projection   (13:199;25:365)

195. It is important for the nurse to understand that Mr. Smith's hypertension is

   A. a substitute for his anger
   B. a symptom of his anger
   C. an expression of his anger
   D. a defense against his anger   (21:347)

Questions 196 to 199

Mr. Hafer, a prominent businessman, has been admitted to the hospital for a bleeding ulcer.

196. The main conflict of a person with a peptic ulcer is thought to be between the

   A. id vs. ego and superego
   B. id vs. superego
   C. ego vs. superego
   D. id and ego vs. superego   (20:459)

197. Which statement most accurately expresses Mr. Hafer's basic conflict?

   A. "Leave the Maalox here and I'll take it myself."
   B. "I could take my Maalox every hour if you will leave it here, but I'd prefer that you give it to me."
   C. "No, you bring it to me when I should take it, you're in charge."
   D. "That stuff tastes terrible. I won't take it."   (20:459)

198. Which of the following statements concerning the incidence of peptic ulcer is/are true?

   a. it occurs more commonly in men than in women
   b. it is commonly seen in persons subject to depression
   c. it is commonly seen in persons subject to alcoholism
   d. it is commonly seen in schizophrenics

   A. a only
   B. b and c
   C. a, b, and c
   D. a and d   (20:459)

199. While caring for patients with a psychophysiological problem, such as ulcers, the nurse should understand that

   A. good nursing care of the physical symptoms will decrease the emotional conflict
   B. it is important to help the patient repress his underlying feelings
   C. there is a good chance that the emotional conflict will lessen as the physical symptoms lessen
   D. a threat to emotional security will lead to an increase in physiological symptoms   (20:459)

D. Depressive Reactions

Directions: For each of the following multiple choice questions, select the ONE most appropriate answer.

200. Depression can be described as

    a. a normal or abnormal mood state which may accompany any psychiatric disorder
    b. a syndrome or symptom complex
    c. a disease process
    d. a complex of psychodynamic mechanisms

    A. a and b
    B. a, b, and c
    C. a, b, c, and d
    D. c and d   (25:174–85)

201. Which of the following statements about depression are true?

    a. it is more common in married individuals
    b. it is more common in men
    c. it is more frequent in the middle-aged and elderly
    d. it is more frequent in southern blacks than northern blacks

    A. a and c
    B. b and c
    C. a and d
    D. b and d   (6:III:75–6)

202. Which of the following are cognitive signs or symptoms of depression?

    a. low self-evaluation
    b. sadness or apathy
    c. increased dependency
    d. indecisiveness

    A. a and d
    B. b and c
    C. a, b, and c
    D. b, c, and d   (6:III:62)

203. Basic physiological signs of depression include all of the following *except*

    A. anorexia
    B. constipation
    C. insomnia
    D. dry mouth   (21:231)

204. All of the following statements about endogenous depression are true *except* that they

    A. are relatively unaffected by external events
    B. usually present a more severe or psychotic picture than exogenous depressions
    C. are often referred to as neurotic or reactive depressions
    D. are usually the result of biological or constitutionally determined patterns
                                  (25:181–82)

205. Which of the following statements regarding depression are true?

    a. the loss of a loved object is the most common precipitant of depression
    b. depression is a result of defensive processes interfering with the normal progress of the mourning process
    c. a child is particularly vulnerable to loss, and thus depression, from 6 months to 4 years of age
    d. Reneé Spitz has shown that marasmus is the extreme result of anaclitic depression in infants with gross neglect

    A. a and b
    B. c and d
    C. a, b, and c
    D. a, b, c, and d   (25:182;20:538–39)

Directions: MATCH the following numbered description with the letter which indicates the correct label according to Freudian theory regarding the psychodynamics of mourning and depression.

Questions 206 to 211

206. Loss or separation from a loved one (20:56)
207. Hypercathexis of the lost object   (1:99)

208. Profoundly painful dejection   (1:98–9)
209. Reattachment of the libido onto a new object
        (1:99)
210. Repetitive self-reproaches with lack of feelings of shame   (25:181)
211. Introjection and identification of the ego
with the lost object   (32:20–1)

    A.   Mourning
    B.   Depression
    C.   Both mourning and depression

Directions: For each of the following multiple choice questions, select the ONE most appropriate answer.

Questions 212 to 216

Jane Carol, the wife of a successful business executive and mother of two small children ages four and six, suddenly finds herself a widow due to her husband John's death in a plane crash.

212. The most common initial reaction of Jane's on hearing this news would be

    A.   to burst into tears and sob uncontrollably
    B.   to react with anger toward the person who tells her of John's death
    C.   to respond with denial, "Oh no, I don't believe it."
    D.   to withdraw and experience a kind of disorganization   (13:236)

213. Jane is concerned with how to tell her two young children about their father's death. Which of the following is the most appropriate initial action on Jane's part?

    A.   to send the children to a close relative's home until after the funeral
    B.   to explain to the children that "Daddy has had to be away longer than he expected on business."
    C.   to tell the children that Daddy died in a plane crash and that Mommy is very sad

    D.   to sit down and calmly explain to the children that life is unpredictable and that each of us will die at some point   (13:247–48)

214. During the three to six weeks following the funeral, Jane's friends find it difficult to know how to behave toward Jane who has become increasingly withdrawn and isolated. Which of the following actions would be most therapeutic for Jane?

    A.   leave Jane alone and allow her privacy in her mourning
    B.   make a special effort to encourage Jane to become involved again in social activities
    C.   encourage Jane to verbalize her feelings about John's death and her memories of their life together
    D.   encourage Jane to move to a new community and find a challenging job   (13:244)

215. All of the following behaviors would be considered part of the normal mourning process *except*

    A.   extreme feelings of sadness and dejection
    B.   loss of interest in her usual activities
    C.   decrease in self esteem and repetitive self-reproaches
    D.   loss of capacity to express love   (25:183–84)

216. If Jane is unable to work through the normal mourning process and goes into a clinical depression, which of the following defense mechanisms is utilized?

    A.   denial
    B.   introjection
    C.   repression
    D.   suppression   (25:185–86)

217. The classic observations of acute grief reactions following the 1943 Coconut Grove nightclub fire were made by

    A.   Erich Lindemann
    B.   John Bowlby
    C.   Gerald Caplan
    D.   Elizabeth Kubler-Ross   (32:10–11)

218. Which of the following might illustrate the concept of object loss?

    a. one's reaction to the death of a spouse

    b. one's reaction to the loss of a job

    c. one's reaction to menopause

    d. one's reaction to a forced retirement

A. a only

B. b and d

C. a, b, and d

D. a, b, c, and d   (13:236–37)

219. The characteristic which differentiates a pathological mourning process (depression) from a normal mourning process is a

A. loss of interest in the external world

B. loss of capacity to love

C. feeling of sadness and despair

D. lowering of self-esteem   (25:181)

220. Mr. Green, a depressed client, is uneasy about attending ward activities. Miss Peters, the nurse, explains the ward routine to Mr. Green, emphasizing quiet non-competitive activities. There is a movie scheduled on the unit. Miss Peters is most likely to help Mr. Green attend the movie if she says

A. "Mr. Green, I'll be back to take you to the movies in an hour."

B. "Mr. Green, there's a movie this afternoon. I'm sure it will cheer you up."

C. "Mr. Green, it's up to you, but there's a movie you might attend."

D. "You'd like to go to the movie, wouldn't you?"   (13:264)

221. In planning ward activities for the depressed patient, the most appropriate intervention in the early stages of hospitalization would be

A. assigning menial tasks

B. providing a minimal routine of activities

C. assigning a regular schedule of activities

D. allowing a choice of activities (2:131–33)

222. The best time to encourage the depressed patient to participate in occupational and recreational activities is

A. early in the morning

B. late afternoon or early evening

C. following electroshock therapy

D. when his interest begins to appear
    (21:231–32)

223. All of the following are symptoms of depression *except*

A. dry mouth, hypochondriacal complaints, increase in appetite

B. constipation, amenorrhea, early morning awakening

C. headaches, digestive disturbances, angry outbursts

D. withdrawal from social situations, fatigue, slowness of movements (20:111)

224. In caring for the depressed client who expresses the belief that he does not deserve to eat, the nurse would

A. wait until the client desires food

B. tell him that food is part of his care

C. serve him his food in his room

D. remain with him and quietly encourage him   (10:194)

Questions 225 to 230

Nancy Backer is a 38-year-old, extremely excitable woman who frequently laughs, shouts, and runs about the ward. She is meddlesome and domineering with other patients and frequently offers to assist the staff in their duties.

225. The nurse caring for Miss Backer needs to understand that

A. such activity, if not curtailed, could lead to extreme physical exhaustion

B. fatigue from the day's activities will probably help Miss Backer sleep better at night

C. Miss Backer should be given large amounts of food to compensate for energy lost in activity

D. Miss Backer will stop this behavior when her physiological needs become great   (2:136)

226. The aspect of Miss Backer's care which the nurse needs to be most concerned with is

    A. skin care
    B. elimination
    C. nutrition
    D. diversion   (2:143)

227. Miss Backer goes up to other patients, interrupts what they are doing, asks them questions, and then goes on before they can answer. Which action by the nurse would be most helpful?

    A. suggest that she read the daily newspaper to an older patient
    B. restrict the number of patients to whom she has access
    C. explain that she may have to be sent to another ward unless she can stop annoying others
    D. suggest that she speak only when spoken to   (2:142)

228. Miss Backer continues to be overactive and unable to concentrate on any one subject for more than a few minutes. Which action by the nurse would probably be of most help to Miss Backer?

    A. enforce rest periods in her room
    B. reduce external stimuli to a minimum
    C. tactfully suggest that she participate in all ward activities
    D. tactfully suggest that she avoid planned ward activities   (2:142)

229. Later, in planning activities for Miss Backer, it would be most appropriate for the nurse to

    A. put her in charge of a patient group in order to constructively channel her activities
    B. keep her from assuming more responsibility than she can handle
    C. solicit her suggestions for planning ward activities
    D. suggest activities requiring mental concentration in order to limit physical activity   (2:142)

230. Which group of occupational therapy projects would be most suitable for an overactive patient like Miss Backer?

    A. loom weaving, finger painting, and needlepoint
    B. making ceramic pottery, binding books, and making artificial flowers
    C. tearing rags for rugs, pounding metal for ash trays, and washing walls
    D. beadweaving, clay modeling, and oil painting   (2:140–41)

231. Which body and temperament types have been correlated with manic-depressive disorders?

    A. athletic type—extrovert
    B. asthenic type—extrovert
    C. pyknic type—extrovert
    D. pyknic type—ambivert   (26:119)

232. The usual age of onset for manic depressive psychosis is

    A. 15 to 25 years
    B. 35 to 50 years
    C. 20 to 35 years
    D. over 45 years   (6:III:462)

233. The nurse would expect the manic patient to respond unfavorably to

    a. postponement of activities
    b. substitution of activities
    c. competitive activities
    d. supervision of activities

    A. a, b, and d
    B. a and c
    C. c only
    D. b and d   (2:140–41)

234. Which of the following activities is most suitable for the manic patient?

    a. tearing cloth for rag rugs
    b. raking leaves
    c. knitting
    d. jigsaw puzzles

    A. a and b
    B. b and c
    C. a, d, and c
    D. a, b, c, and d   (2:141)

235. Which activity would be most appropriate for a manic client?

A. chess
B. scrabble
C. needlepoint
D. writing   (2:141)

236. Mrs. Calvin is talking with the nurse. She says, "My, I enjoy babies. They're so little, like dolls. Did you see Carol Channing sing 'Hello, Dolly', I guess blondes do have more fun." This is an example of

A. rambling
B. word salad
C. flight of ideas
D. circumstantiality   (20:103)

Questions 237 to 241

Mrs. Brennan was admitted to the hospital two days ago with a diagnosis of manic-depressive psychosis. She is very hyperactive and in report this A.M. the nurse learns that Mrs. Brennan has not slept since admission.

237. On entering the Day Room, the nurse finds Mrs. Brennan dancing to loud radio music. Her most appropriate response to Mrs. Brennan would be

A. "Mrs. Brennan, please turn the radio down so we can hear ourselves talk."
B. "Mrs. Brennan, you and I had planned to talk together this morning. Let's go to your room."
C. "Mrs. Brennan, how are you ever going to get any rest if you keep that music on?"
D. "Mrs. Brennan, do you think you could sit still for a few minutes so we can talk?"   (10:194)

238. Mrs. Brennan ignores the nurse, continues dancing and begins to complain vociferously. The nurse's primary concern at this point should be that

A. Mrs. Brennan had not remembered their scheduled appointment
B. Mrs. Brennan may be nearing the point of physical exhaustion

C. Mrs. Brennan's behavior is disruptive to the whole ward
D. Mrs. Brennan is ignoring her overtures to make contact   (10:184)

239. The nurse decides to contact the doctor-on-call for a medication order. The most appropriate medication at this time for Mrs. Brennan would be

A. thorozine 100 mg P.O.
B. thorazine 25 mg I.M.
C. lithonate 200 mg P.O.
D. lithonate 50 mg I.M.   (20:623–25)

240. The psychodynamic explanation of the manic behavior of a manic-depressive patient is that the mania is a

A. projection of the basic id impulses
B. denial of the underlying depression
C. suppression of feelings of sadness due to loss
D. sublimation for socially unacceptable feelings   (20:378)

241. The overactive behavior demonstrated by a catatonic patient differs from that of a manic patient in that the catatonic patient

A. may smile or laugh inappropriately while speaking of very disturbing thoughts
B. appears to have boundless energy
C. appears elated and talks excessively
D. frequently expresses ideas of grandeur   (28:163)

242. All of the following statements about the epidemiology of manic-depressive psychosis are true *except*

A. the incidence of manic-depressive psychoses is significantly higher in the United States than in England and Wales
B. there are some studies which indicate that manic-depressive psychosis is seen more frequently in higher social classes
C. some patients diagnosed as manic-depressive exhibit only recurrent depressions

D. a sibling of a manic-depressive has 25 times higher chance of becoming manic-depressive than the average individual (20:366)

Questions 243 to 244

Mrs. Moore is extremely restless, physically overactive, and irritable. She is easily distracted by persons or events in her environment and expends a great deal of energy flitting from one activity to another. She "takes over" for other patients and is interfering. She is sarcastic and supercilious toward staff.

243. Mrs. Moore's behavior serves all of the following purposes *except*

A. an outlet for tension
B. a defense against emotions she feels
C. a means of maintaining her superior feelings
D. a means of maintaining peer relationships (10:184)

244. A group of student nurses comes to the unit. Mrs. Moore approaches them and says, "What are you gaping at? Do you think that we're all crazy? What kind of place do you think this is?" Understanding the dynamics of Mrs. Moore might lead the students to recognize all of the following *except*

A. Mrs. Moore reacts to her new stimuli in an exaggerated fashion in order to maintain her security
B. Mrs. Moore seeks to embarrass others in an attempt to externalize hostility
C. Mrs. Moore will continue to pursue this topic as she cannot easily change the focus of her attention
D. Mrs. Moore neither wants nor expects an answer, but is simply attempting to keep others at a safe distance (10:184)

245. In working with the client who is overactive, the nurse would indicate awareness of his dynamics if she

A. selects a quiet area and responds in a quiet, slow manner

B. selects a quiet area and attempts to focus the client on the conversation
C. isolates the client and limits her own verbal responses
D. suggests the client join a sing-a-long and involve himself in activities (9:148–49)

246. Lithium intoxication symptoms include

A. excessive thirst, polyuria, persistent diarrhea, and vomiting
B. increased salivation, polyuria, persistent diarrhea, and vomiting
C. constipation, dry mouth, and vertigo
D. diarrhea, vomiting, and leukopenia (20:633)

Questions 247 to 252

Mrs. Cassidy is a 50-year-old housewife who was admitted to the hospital because she no longer took any interest in her home or family. Frequently, she would sit for long periods of time slumped in a chair, staring into space. At other times, she paced the hall pulling at her hair, wringing her hands, and crying, "I have sinned." She told the nurse that someone had removed her stomach. Mrs. Cassidy has a history of one suicidal attempt.

247. When Mrs. Cassidy complains that she cannot eat because her stomach has been removed, the nurse should

A. explain that the doctor said her stomach was all right
B. ignore her complaint and change the subject
C. tease her for thinking her stomach is gone
D. listen to her complaint and remind her that her laboratory tests have all been normal (20:361)

248. When Mrs. Cassidy paces up and down the hall, wailing and pulling her hair, she is most likely

A. trying to get attention from the staff
B. fulfilling a need for atonement
C. furious that she has been hospitalized
D. totally unable to control her behavior (20:359)

249. The most appropriate response on the part of the nurse would be to

    A. tell her to stop pacing and talk with other patients
    B. try to interest her in a television program
    C. give her a simple task to do
    D. ask the doctor for an order to seclude her   (2:130–31)

250. When Mrs. Cassidy expresses feelings of unworthiness, the best response on the part of the nurse would be

    A. "I am sure you have led a good life, Mrs. Cassidy."
    B. "Try to forget those thoughts and join our card game."
    C. "Your family loves you very much."
    D. "As you begin to get well, these feelings will disappear."   (2:130)

251. Mrs. Cassidy tells the nurse, "I wish I were dead. I have nothing to live for." The most appropriate response by the nurse would be

    A. "You have lots to live for—a nice home, family, and friends."
    B. "It's too nice a day for such thoughts. Let's go for a walk."
    C. "Have you been thinking about dying?"
    D. "I'll sit here with you and we can talk about something more pleasant."
        (20:362)

252. The danger of another suicidal attempt by Mrs. Cassidy is greatest

    A. during the first week of admission to the hospital
    B. when she is deeply depressed
    C. when she apparently is recovering from her depression
    D. during the periods she is very agitated
        (2:134)

253. The most commonly accepted explanation of involutional psychosis is

    A. hormonal changes of menopause
    B. emotional trauma of this time of life

C. hormonal imbalance
D. crises related to sexual role identity
    (2:124)

254. Mr. Grier tells the nurse, "I don't want to die. See that window? I'm going to jump out!" This is an example of

    A. autism
    B. looseness of association
    C. ambivalence
    D. impulsivity   (10:231)

255. The nurse's most appropriate response to Mr. Grier would be

    A. "I'll stay with you, Mr. Grier, so you won't hurt yourself."
    B. "You cannot jump out the window, Mr. Grier."
    C. "Would you like me to stay with you, Mr. Grier?"
    D. "Why would you want to kill yourself, Mr. Grier?"   (10:201;34:191)

Questions 256 to 257

Mrs. Klein is a 40-year-old woman who became severly depressed after the birth of her fourth child. The baby caused physical and emotional strain as well as a financial burden on the family. Although she talked about her happiness in having a baby, she also had thoughts indicating her wish not to have a baby.

256. Mrs. Klein is exhibiting

    A. ambivalent feelings
    B. her need to be independent
    C. ambivalent feelings and realistic guilt
    D. rejection of the maternal role   (4:9)

257. In planning care for Mrs. Klein, the nurse should

    A. encourage Mrs. Klein to assume care for the new baby
    B. point out the reality of the situation
    C. help her to bear the painful feelings causing the guilt
    D. reinforce her need to be a good person   (10:133)

258. Which of the following symptoms are seen as indications of depression in latency-aged children?

    a. temper tantrums
    b. boredom
    c. accident proneness
    d. crying

    A. a and b
    B. c and d
    C. a and c
    D. b and d   (18:108)

259. Persistence of which of the following traits in adolescents indicates depression?

    A. boredom
    B. restlessness
    C. an inability to be alone
    D. all of the above   (6:II:296)

260. Factors that increase the suicidal risk during adolescence include

    A. sexual acting out
    B. broken homes
    C. cultural influences
    D. all of the above   (18:107–08)

261. Which of the following treatments is most useful for the client who is a continual suicidal risk even in a psychiatric hospital?

    A. tricyclic compounds
    B. monoamine oxidase inhibitors
    C. electroshock therapy
    D. lithium   (2:127–28)

262. Which of the following factors has been most successful in reducing the suicide rate among hospitalized suicidal patients?

    A. restricting the patients from possessing articles like shoelaces, belts, razors
    B. the introduction of electroshock therapy
    C. the newer psychoactive drugs
    D. the "open-door" policy and emphasis on a therapeutic interpersonal milieu
                    (6:III:760)

263. At which point is the risk of suicide greatest in depressed hospitalized patients?

    a. during hospitalization
    b. during weekend leaves
    c. immediately before discharge
    d. shortly after discharge

    A. a and b
    B. c and d
    C. b and d
    D. a and c   (6:III:67)

264. Which of the following is the *least* accurate belief about suicide?

    A. suicide is more common in urban slum areas than in suburbs
    B. suicide seldom happens without some type of warning
    C. improvement after a depressive episode probably means the suicide risk is over
    D. people who talk about suicide frequently attempt suicide   (32:25–31)

E. Schizophrenia

Directions: For each of the following multiple choice questions, select the ONE most appropriate answer.

265. A functional psychosis implies

    A. a favorable prognosis
    B. organic impairment
    C. psychogenic origin
    D. an unfavorable prognosis   (10:412)

266. The term "schizophrenia" refers to

    A. breaking up of normal syntheses of thought, feeling, and activity in one individual
    B. appearance of more than one distinct set of personality traits in one individual
    C. apparent splitting of the activities of the mind from those of the body of one individual
    D. physiological disjunction of the limbic system from the cerebrum within the brain   (4:86)

267. Primary symptoms of schizophrenia include

    a. delusions
    b. loosening of association
    c. autism
    d. disturbances of affect

    A. a and b
    B. a, b, and c
    C. b, c, and d
    D. a, b, c, and d   (20:310–11)

268. Accessory (secondary) symptoms of schizophrenia include

    a. hallucinations
    b. delusions
    c. catatonic phenomena
    d. incongruous affect

    A. a and b
    B. a, b, and c
    C. a, b, c, and d
    D. a, c, and d   (20:311)

269. The classic four types of schizophrenia are considered to be

    A. basic subdivisions
    B. unchangeable
    C. descriptive
    D. prognostically significant   (2:103–04)

270. The most *commonly* held theory about the etiology of schizophrenia is that schizophrenia

    A. results from defective genes
    B. is caused by a biochemical abnormality
    C. results from abnormal family communication patterns
    D. is caused by an interaction of environmental and organic influences   (21:267)

271. Biological factors which are thought to be of significance in the etiology of schizophrenia include

    a. genetic predisposition
    b. constitutional weakness
    c. immunological disorder
    d. metabolic disturbance

    A. a and b
    B. a, b, and c
    C. a and c
    D. a, b, c, and d   (20:312–15)

272. Which of the following are typical features of schizophrenia?

    a. free association
    b. denial of reality
    c. preoccupation with one's fantasies
    d. contradictory feelings toward objects and experiences

    A. a, b, and c
    B. b, c, and d
    C. a and b
    D. all of the above   (20:310–11)

273. Experiential factors that have possible significance in the etiology of schizophrenia include

    a. disordered parental relationships
    b. maternal deprivation or inadequate mothering during the oral stage of development
    c. repeated exposure to "double bind" situations
    d. lack of experience with consensual validation

    A. a, b, and c
    B. b, c, and d
    C. b and d
    D. a, b, c, and d   (20:316–17)

274. Process schizophrenia is characterized by the presence of which of the following factors?

    a. blunted affect
    b. insidious onset
    c. massive hallucinatory experiences
    d. sudden onset

    A. a and b
    B. c and d
    C. a and d
    D. b and c   (4:87)

275. The interpersonal theory of schizophrenia is a major contribution of

A. Harry Stack Sullivan
B. Sigmund Freud
C. Eugen Bleuler
D. Carl Rogers   (6:III:633)

276. Prodromal signs of schizophrenia include

A. shyness, aloofness, and anxiety
B. aloofness, introversion, and fastidiousness
C. withdrawal, unhappiness, and lack of ambition
D. shyness, conscientiousness, and anxiety
(20:319)

277. Which of the following describe the nature of ambivalence in the schizophrenic client?

a. there is ambivalence of impulse, idea, and affect
b. ambivalence may explain some of the impulsive behavior
c. ambivalent feelings are only present toward highly significant persons and situations
d. ambivalence is present but mainly in regard to thoughts

A. a and b
B. b and c
C. a and d
D. c and d   (20:327:328)

278. Autism is *best* defined as

A. a highly personalized form of thinking
B. a type of mental illness
C. a symptom of psychotic behavior
D. an ego defense mechanism   (10:231–32)

279. Social isolation of the schizophrenic may lead to

a. reduced awareness of perceptual stimulation
b. preoccupation with thought processes
c. regressive infantile thinking processes
d. a decrease in hallucinatory satisfactions

A. a and d
B. a and c

C. a, b, and c
D. b, c, and d   (20:350)

280. Which of the following statements about mothers of schizophrenic clients is true?

A. the majority of mothers are cold, rejecting, or overprotective
B. the majority of mothers are unable to give to their children in a maternal way
C. mothers of schizophrenics seem to play a more directly causative role than fathers
D. there is insufficient evidence to support the concept of a schizophrenogenic mother   (6:III:554–55)

Directions: MATCH the following numbered items with the most appropriate lettered items.

Questions 281 to 285

281. Schismatic family   (14:128)
282. Pseudomutuality   (6:I:187)
283. Mystification   (6:I:187)
284. Double-bind   (6:I:189)
285. Scapegoating   (14:128)

A. Bateson
B. Lidz
C. Laing
D. Bell and Vogel
E. Wynne

Directions: For each of the following multiple choice questions, select the ONE most appropriate answer.

286. Symbiotic involvements in the family can be seen to have origins in

a. a disturbed marital relationship in parents
b. a disturbed marital relationship in grandparents
c. a physiological complication of pregnancy
d. the birth of a sibling

A. a and b
B. a only
C. a and c
D. a and d   (30:125)

287. Childhood schizophrenia is usually characterized by

    A. abrupt onset
    B. delusions and hallucinations
    C. catatonic symptoms
    D. speech disturbances   (2:108)

288. Which of the following factors play a role in the etiology of schizophrenia?

    a. genetic or hereditary factors
    b. perceptual difficulties
    c. environmental stress
    d. neurological disturbance

    A. a and c
    B. a, c, and d
    C. b and c
    D. a, b, c, and d   (20:338–41)

289. Which of the following statements about childhood schizophrenia is *not* accurate?

    A. the primary symptoms are identical to those of adult schizophrenia
    B. many experts differentiate childhood schizophrenia from infantile autism
    C. the link between childhood schizophrenia and adult schizophrenia is uncertain
    D. seclusiveness is recognized as a usual symptom by many authorities   (6:II:86–8)

290. All of the following are symptomatic of infantile autism *except*

    A. experiences panic at separation from the mother
    B. much more interested in mechanical objects than people
    C. extreme solitude evident from early infancy
    D. often appears to be deaf   (6:II:89–90)

291. Billy, age seven, hits John, another patient on a unit for disturbed children. Miss Turner, the nurse, demonstrates understanding of the situation if she

    A. criticizes the act
    B. withdraws her friendly attention
    C. disciplines him in front of John
    D. removes privileges for a week (2:461–62)

292. In working with the schizophrenic patient, the nurse *initially* needs to demonstrate

    A. acceptance
    B. warmth
    C. self-acceptance
    D. tolerance   (10:17)

293. Systematized delusions are characteristic of

    A. paranoia
    B. paranoid schizophrenia
    C. manic depressive psychosis
    D. involutional psychosis   (20:387)

294. If the schizophrenic patient is delusional, his delusions tend to be

    a. extravagant and bizarre
    b. an attempt to problem-solve
    c. specific to his needs
    d. around themes of persecution

    A. a and b
    B. a, b, and c
    C. c and d
    D. a, b, c, and d   (20:325–26)

295. A patient's expression of delusional content serves as a communication in that it

    A. often is a daydream that is treated as if it were real
    B. can be easily grasped if seen as a metaphor
    C. is often a clear analogy to the real situation
    D. is usually related to the environmental stimuli   (20:105–06)

296. Examples of thought disorders include

    a. circumstantiality
    b. automatic knowing
    c. scattering
    d. rationalization

A. a, b, and c
B. a, c, and d
C. b, c, and d
D. a, b, and d   (9:12–15)

297. Which of the following symptoms is *always* present in schizophrenia?

A.. hallucinations
B. delusions
C. fragmentation of thought
D. interpersonal withdrawal   (2:101–02)

298. The most common form of hallucinations in schizophrenia is

A. auditory
B. tactile
C. visual
D. gustatory   (6:III:539)

299. Which of the following physical problems is found in acutely ill patients in catatonic stupor?

A. hypersalivation
B. urinary retention
C. hyperglycemia
D. polyurea   (2:117)

300. According to Peplau, the levels of consciousness in loneliness versus aloneness are most similar to those of

A. projection versus introjection
B. repression versus suppression
C. hallucinations versus delusions
D. negativism versus resistance   (27:II:56)

301. Persecutory delusions can be explained as defense mechanisms which

a. explain the person's failures
b. absolve one from blame for the inability to adjust
c. project one's own intense feelings of hatred
d. are compensatory in nature

A. a and d
B. a and c
C. b and c
D. a, b, and c   (26:452)

302. Which of the following drives are central in the etiology of paranoid disorders?

a. repressed homosexual drives
b. power drives
c. dependency drives
d. affiliative drives

A. a and b
B. b and c
C. a, b, and c
D. b, c, and d   (26:451)

303. One would expect the client to be less delusional and hallucinatory if the client has

A. a feeling of relatedness to others
B. the symptom called to his attention
C. minimal external stimulation
D. an above average intellectual capacity
                                   (18:312–14)

304. Catatonic schizophrenia is *best* characterized by

A. alterations in activity, negativism, automatism, mutism
B. neologisms, withdrawal, regression, suspiciousness
C. ideas of reference, superciliousness, silliness, rage
D. silliness, bizarre delusions, regression, mannerisms   (20:332–34)

305. The hebephrenic type of schizophrenia is *best* characterized by

A. silliness, giggling, bizarre delusions, mannerisms
B. neologism, withdrawal, regression, suspiciousness
C. silliness, hyperactivity, ideas of reference, apathy
D. apathy, fixed delusions, blunt affect, regression   (4:87)

306. Which of the following statements about catatonic excitement are accurate?

 a. the excitement phase is usually related to external stimuli
 b. the patient often seems enraged and may be destructive
 c. there is unorganized and aggressive motor activity
 d. negativism is decreased

 A. a and b
 B. b and c
 C. a and d
 D. c and d   (20:333–34)

307. The preoccupation with the belief that one is being harmed by others is typical of

 A. derealization
 B. delusions of persecution
 C. idea of reference
 D. autistic thinking   (20:106)

Questions 308 to 313

Mary is an above-average student and was her class' valedictorian. She recently began college at a large, highly competitive university. She became disorganized which resulted in failing grades, and her roommate found her sitting in her room, staring and unresponsive. When this persisted for 24 hours, Mary's parents were contacted and they admitted her to the psychiatric ward of the general hospital.

308. Mary's illness can best be seen as related to a need for

 A. security, comfort, and protection
 B. parental guidance
 C. peer support
 D. continued academic achievement
                                (10:132)

309. Mary is observed by the nurse who notes that Mary is remaining in one area most of the day and only moves when she is guided to another area. This behavior is an example of

 A. negativism
 B. waxy flexibility

 C. echopraxia
 D. stupor   (20:333)

310. Mary avoids the nurse for two weeks. She stays in the bathroom or lies on her bed, feigning sleep. The nurse recognizes that this behavior indicates

 A. a rejection of the nurse by Mary
 B. a negative transference towards the nurse
 C. coping behavior on the part of Mary
 D. Mary's unwillingness to seek help
                                (20:333)

311. One day, Mary says to the nurse, "They are telling me I am going crazy." She appears to be listening intently. The nurse indicates an understanding of Mary's behavior by responding

 A. "Do they say this often, Mary?"
 B. "I don't hear anything, Mary. Tell me how you feel."
 C. "Why do they say that, Mary?"
 D. "Let's talk about something else."
                                (18:373)

312. Which would be most helpful to Mary initially?

 A. to encourage her to relate to other clients
 B. to encourage her to participate in activities
 C. to allow her to be alone when she wishes
 D. to accept her limited verbal communication
                                (18:306)

313. Mary is probably experiencing

 A. a psychotic disorder
 B. separation anxiety
 C. a depressive reaction
 D. a mood disorder   (4:81)

314. Mrs. Cochran expresses the belief that the F.B.I. is out to kill her. In caring for her, the nurse should recognize that Mrs. Cochran

 a. will probably see the nurses and doctors as protectors
 b. may interpret the hospital and its routines as threatening

c. may react impulsively out of fear

d. will correct her thinking after the doctor has spoken to her

A. a and c

B. b and d

C. b and c

D. a, b, c, and d (27:II:23–24)

315. If a patient states, "The voices tell me that I should not talk with you," the nurse's best response would be

A. "Do they say why you shouldn't?"

B. "Those voices are only in your head."

C. "When do they say this?"

D. "I don't hear them but can we talk about how you are feeling now?" (10:244–45;34:186–87)

316. Mrs. Cook, a catatonic schizophrenic, comes into the lounge and begins to recite obscenities. The nurse, Mrs. Potter, can best assist Mrs. Cook in a therapeutic manner if she

A. allows Mrs. Cook to continue without comment

B. asks Mrs. Cook to please stop her behavior

C. escorts Mrs. Cook gently to her room to talk

D. waits for the group to limit Mrs. Cook's behavior (21:463)

317. Mr. Jackson is diagnosed as paranoid schizophrenic. He is to have routine admission blood work and x-rays. Which verbal approach by the nurse would indicate the best understanding of Mr. Jackson's psychodynamics?

A. "Mr. Jackson, the hospital requires all clients to have certain blood tests and x-rays. I will take you now."

B. "Mr. Jackson, we are trying to help you and will be doing some tests on you."

C. "Mr. Jackson, I am going to take you to the treatment room for some tests. It's part of your therapy."

D. "Mr. Jackson, I know it's unpleasant, but you need to go for some tests now." (10:252)

318. Mr. Hill is a suspicious client. Mr. Gannon, a staff nurse, has initiated a relationship with Mr. Hill. They have been meeting for one-half hour, three times a week. During the second week, Mr. Hill tells him that all of the other clients dislike him. Mr. Gannon's best initial response would be

A. "Can you give me an example? I'm not certain I know what you mean."

B. "Mr. Hill, perhaps you don't give them a chance."

C. "It's only been 2 weeks since you came; it takes time to get to know people."

D. "I'll bring this up tomorrow at our daily meeting." (34:201)

Questions 319 to 320

Mr. Thomas is a 33-year-old laborer who is admitted to the emergency room due to assaultive behavior. He has many paranoid delusions and threatens to fight his way out of the hospital. He has been certified.

319. The nurse should

A. call additional staff to admit Mr. Thomas

B. use restraints so that he cannot hurt others

C. reason with Mr. Thomas

D. be friendly and attempt to persuade him to stay (31:47)

320. The nurse is ready to bring Mr. Thomas to the ward. The most appropriate comment would be

A. "Mr. Thomas, we are going to take you to the unit now."

B. "Mr. Thomas, you'll only be on the unit a few days. No one will hurt you."

C. "Mr. Thomas, I know you're upset, but you'll feel differently when you see the unit."

D. "Mr. Thomas, your family decided you need to be hospitalized. They realize you're upset." (31:47)

Questions 321 to 323

Mrs. Adams, a 25-year-old housewife is admitted to the hospital with a diagnosis of schizophrenia, catatonic type. She is brought to the hospital on a stretcher, does not respond to questioning, and appears to be reacting to voices. She passively assumes and maintains the positions she is placed in while being dressed.

321. Which of the following statements about patients in a catatonic stupor is *in*correct?

   A. they may exhibit extreme negativism
   B. their posture frequently has symbolic meanings
   C. they are unaware of their external surroundings
   D. they may have hallucinations and delusions   (26:433)

322. Mrs. Adams appears to be responding to voices. She cries out at intervals, "No, no, I didn't kill him!" After one of these episodes, she turns to the nurse and states, "You know the truth, tell that policeman. Please help me." Which of the following would be the best response on the part of the nurse?

   A. "Mrs. Adams, I want to help you. I don't hear a policeman, but this must frighten you very much."
   B. to sit with Mrs. Adams and not respond verbally to her statements since talking about her experience may upset her more
   C. "Mrs. Adams, do not become so upset. No one is talking to you as we are alone. This is part of your illness."
   D. "Who are they saying you killed, Mrs. Adams?"   (10:243–45)

323. The ambivalence and indecision in the catatonic patient can best be handled by

   A. allowing Mrs. Adams to make all minor decisions while the staff makes the major decisions for her
   B. planning a strict regime for Mrs. Adams to which she must adhere, thus freeing her of decision-making

   C. limiting group participation and activity in an effort to protect Mrs. Adams from conflicting situations where decisions are necessary
   D. permitting Mrs. Adams to make decisions and supporting these decisions when they do not endanger herself or others   (13:301–06)

324. Mr. Garson is talking with the nurse. He says to her, "Am I schizophrenic?" The most therapeutic response would be

   A. "Why do you ask, Mr. Garson?"
   B. "Can you tell me what brought that to mind, Mr. Garson?"
   C. "You'll have to ask your doctor, Mr. Garson. He makes the diagnosis."
   D. "We do not diagnose people, Mr. Garson."   (10:100)

Questions 325 to 327

Mr. Clemson is playing cards with two student nurses and another patient. He begins pulling on his ear. One of the student nurses asks, "Is your ear bothering you, Mr. Clemson?" Mr. Clemson replies, "Yes, it's those radios he put in my ear. You know all about it."

325. The most appropriate response from the student would be

   A. "When did this happen, Mr. Clemson?"
   B. "You think I know all about it?"
   C. "Who put radios in your ear?"
   D. "Why would someone do that?"   (10:245)

326. Mr. Clemson's statement can best be described as

   A. an hallucination
   B. a delusion
   C. an illusion
   D. an idea of reference   (10:233)

327. In working with Mr. Clemson, the nurse needs to attempt to

   A. understand what his behavior represents
   B. interpret Mr. Clemson's behavior

C. limit Mr. Clemson's expression of psychopathology

D. avoid meeting the covert needs expressed (27:II:23)

Questions 328 to 332

Jim Jensen is a 25-year-old male patient on an admission ward. Much of the time, he appears disheveled, and he tends to sit in the same position for long periods of time.

328. Mr. Jensen is sitting in a corner of the ward, head down and unresponsive. Which assumption by the nurse about Mr. Jensen is *most* justified?

A. he is unaware of what is going on around him

B. he may be aware of what is going on around him

C. he is afraid to show that he is interested in what is going on

D. he is uninterested in what is going on (2:109)

329. When the nurse approaches Mr. Jensen, he walks away. Which initial interpretation of this behavior by the nurse is *most* justified?

A. he is "asking" to be pursued

B. he believes he has no nursing needs

C. he had had previous experiences that make him distrust nurses

D. he expects no satisfaction from this relationship (2:119)

330. After several weeks on the unit, Mr. Jensen tends to remain with the nurse but does not respond to her attempts at communication. The concept that would be most helpful in planning effective nursing care is

A. securing information from the patient is a major responsibility of the nurse

B. a therapeutic relationship can be established without conversation

C. patients should be encouraged to be physically active as a substitute for socialization

D. verbal exchange is necessary in establishing a positive relationship (2:380)

331. Which action by the nurse would be most appropriate in helping Mr. Jensen to communicate verbally?

A. ask him questions until he is stimulated to respond

B. greet him and talk continuously to him until he responds

C. greet him, make occasional comments and continue, if he responds

D. speak to him only if he initiates the conversation (2:390)

332. Which comment by the nurse is most appropriate in encouraging Mr. Jensen to go outdoors for a walk?

A. "Are you going out with the group today, Mr. Jensen?"

B. "Come on everyone, let's go for a walk."

C. "Let's go for a walk, Mr. Jensen."

D. "Do you mind joining the group for a walk, Mr. Jensen?" (2:112–31)

333. Stanton and Schwartz demonstrated that patient behavior, such as unexplained excitement in a chronic schizophrenic patient, can be related to

A. length of hospitalization

B. the professional status of staff members

C. covert conflict between staff members

D. the psychopathology of the patient group (6:III:29)

334. Paul is an adolescent whose mother encourages him to socialize more, yet when he suggests going out to meet people, his mother tells him that she does not feel well and needs his help. This can *best* be described as

A. inconsistent and ambivalent behavior

B. a "double-bind" transaction

C. conflicting communication

D. maternal overprotection (4:30)

335. In talking with the suspicious patient, the nursing behavior that is *most* helpful is one that is

    A. matter-of-fact, honest, and consistent
    B. honest, consistent, and intellectual
    C. matter-of-fact, honest, with physical closeness
    D. consistent, honest, with physical closeness (26:456–57)

Questions 336 to 339

Miss Scala, a staff nurse, is talking with the doctor. Afterwards, she starts to go back to the nurses' station. Mr. Clark stops her and says, "That doctor told you I can't go home."

336. The most appropriate response on the part of the nurse would be

    A. "The doctor and I weren't talking about you, Mr. Clark."
    B. "Do you want to go home, Mr. Clark?"
    C. "You saw me talking with the doctor?"
    D. "You'll be going home, Mr. Clark." (10:244)

337. Mr. Clark's belief that Miss Scala and the doctor were talking about him could best be described as

    A. a delusion
    B. an illusion
    C. an idea of reference
    D. a delusion of persecution (10:413)

338. Mr. Clark's doctor prescribes thorazine, 100 mg Q.I.D. A dangerous untoward effect of this medication is

    A. hypertension
    B. parkinsonism
    C. agranulocytosis
    D. somnolence (20:626)

339. Mr. Clark has been quite angry with another patient and argued with him frequently during the week. He says to Miss Scala, "Are you angry? You look it." Miss Scala indicates her support of Mr. Clark by responding

    A. "No, I'm not angry. Why do you ask?"
    B. "Have you known people to behave a certain way when they're angry?"
    C. "Everyone seems angry to you today, Mr. Clark."
    D. "There is no reason for me to be angry, Mr. Clark." (10:234)

Questions 340 to 341

Miss Jones, 21-years-old, has been admitted to the psychiatric unit. She has been living with her parents and was brought to the hospital by them. They state that she does not leave her room, stares into space, and has not eaten in two days. They also comment that she has always been quiet and is a "good" daughter.

340. The most immediate concerns for nursing care for Miss Jones would be

    a. insure adequate food and fluid intake
    b. approach her at her present level of functioning
    c. observe her behavior
    d. stimulate interest in the environment

    A. a and b
    B. a, b, and c
    C. a, b, c, and d
    D. a and c (2:110–19)

341. Miss Jones is told about the unit routine and is shown to her room. She later appears in the dining room unclothed. The nurse approaches Miss Jones and says

    A. "I will take you to your room Miss Jones, so you can get dressed."
    B. "Miss Jones, please return to your room and get dressed."
    C. "Miss Jones, do you realize you're not dressed?"
    D. "Miss Jones, unless you get dressed, you will have to stay in your room." (27:II:21)

342. The nurse asks Miss Olsen to go to activities. Miss Olsen responds, "She doesn't want to go. She wants to sleep." This response is an example of

    A. a delusional ideation
    B. a feeling of depersonalization
    C. an idea of reference
    D. the use of global pronouns   (4:28)

343. Effective hospital care of the schizophrenic patient occurs when the staff members

    a. provide healthy models for identification
    b. are above average intelligence and education
    c. support rewarding relationships
    d. encourage client verbal communication

    A. a, b, and c
    B. a, c, and d
    C. b, c, and d
    D. a, b, c, and d   (20:348)

344. The fundamental goal of the nurse in caring for the schizophrenic is to

    A. create a safe environment
    B. care for his physical well-being
    C. offer reassuring interpersonal contact
    D. return him to the community   (2:110)

345. In caring for the patient who exhibits poor reality testing, the nurse should

    A. correct the patient's wrong thinking
    B. encourage the expression of autistic material
    C. let the patient know when she does not understand him
    D. change the subject or terminate conversation that is autistic   (10:243)

346. The nurse asks the patient, "What brought you to the hospital?" The patient replies, "A bus!" This is an example of

    A. denial
    B. concreteness of thought
    C. blocking
    D. resistance   (25:234)

347. Three days after admission, Miss Todd's nurse gives the following description of her behavior: "Apparently Miss Todd has slept only for brief periods in the previous 48 hours. She assumes unusual postures and paces around the room in a sterotyped manner. Frequently, she does not appear to respond to auditory and visual stimuli. She has removed all her clothing several times and once attempted to set fire to it. Her affect is flat." These behaviors are most typical of

    A. dissociative reaction
    B. catatonic schizophrenic reaction
    C. hebephrenic schizophrenic reaction
    D. simple schizophrenic reaction   (21:262)

348. In working with a paranoid patient, the nurse should recognize the patient's need for

    A. reassurance
    B. warmth
    C. physical closeness
    D. emotional distance   (34:202)

349. Mr. Clark is suspicious that the nurses are trying to poison him. In giving him medication, it is important that the nurse

    A. not identify the kind of medication
    B. disguise the taste
    C. use parenteral medication if possible
    D. be sure that Mr. Clark swallows it
                                          (2:118)

350. The most important aspect of hospitalization for the schizophrenic client is

    A. well-regulated and structured therapeutic milieu
    B. the one-to-one relationship
    C. the freedom to act "crazy"
    D. presence of professional personnel
                                          (20:351)

351. Which of the following accurately describes the prognosis of schizophrenia?

    A. reactive schizophrenia generally has a less favorable prognosis than process schizophrenia
    B. few patients hospitalized for the first time with acute schizophrenia can be expected to make a "social" recovery
    C. a marked affect component (depression, anxiety, confusion) generally indicates a better prognosis
    D. none of the above   (20:344)

352. The type of schizophrenia with the least favorable prognosis is

    A. catatonic
    B. hebephrenic
    C. paranoid
    D. schizo-affective   (20:331)

353. All of the following are associated with a good prognosis for the schizophrenic patient *except*

    A. insidious onset
    B. confusion
    C. prominent depressive symptoms
    D. feelings of guilt   (32:94)

354. Favorable prognostic factors in schizophrenic reactions include

    A. rapid onset, external precipitating factors, subjective discomfort
    B. insidious onset, early treatment, subjective discomfort
    C. external precipitating factors, insidious onset, early treatment
    D. external precipitating factors, hypochondriasis, lack of subjective discomfort   (20:342, 344)

355. Whitehorn's study concerning conversation with schizophrenic patients demonstrated that to establish contact with a schizophrenic patient the nurse is most successful if she focuses on

    A. the client's life history
    B. the client's problems
    C. the client's day-to-day activities
    D. all of the above   (2:111)

356. In assisting the regressed schizophrenic patient with grooming and hygiene, the nurse should expect that the patient will

    A. respond to verbal suggestions
    B. need active assistance
    C. respond with negativism
    D. be unable to assist himself   (13:314)

357. Humor is considered an inappropriate response on the therapist's part when working with the client who is

    A. suspicious
    B. anxious
    C. angry
    D. antisocial   (25:288)

358. Appropriate techniques by the nurse to engage the schizophrenic client in verbal communication include

    a. listening for cues to subjects of interest to the client
    b. word-construction games such as Scrabble
    c. introducing topics in which the nurse is well-versed
    d. focusing on the feelings of the client

    A. a and b
    B. c and d
    C. a and d
    D. a, b, and c   (26:445)

359. The "listening attitude" as identified by Arieti refers to

    a. a period of expectant listening
    b. the posture assumed by the hallucinating patient
    c. the first stage of the hallucinatory experience
    d. the first stage of an idea of reference

    A. a and b
    B. a and c
    C. a and d
    D. d only   (18:313–14)

360. The term "Social Breakdown Syndrome" was coined in 1962 by the

    A. American Public Health Association
    B. American Psychiatric Association
    C. National Institute of Mental Health
    D. World Health Organization   (6:II:700)

361. The patterns in the Social Breakdown Syndrome include

    A. withdrawal
    B. anger and hostility
    C. withdrawal, anger, and hostility
    D. none of the above   (6:II:700)

362. The Social Breakdown Syndrome is found in

    A. functional psychoses
    B. organic psychoses
    C. mental retardation
    D. all of the above   (6:II:700)

363. The Social Breakdown Syndrome begins most often in

    a. the community
    b. the hospital
    c. an insidious manner
    d. a single, explosive episode

    A. b and c
    B. a and c
    C. b and d
    D. a and d   (6:II:703)

F.   Organic Disorders

Directions: For each of the following multiple choice questions, select the ONE most appropriate answer.

364. All of the following are characteristics of the organic brain syndrome *except*

    A. impairment of orientation, emotional instability
    B. pupillary changes, tremors
    C. habit deterioration, confabulation
    D. good recent memory, poor remote memory   (25:242–46)

365. Which of the following brain syndromes is most responsive to early recognition and treatment?

    A. Pick's Disease
    B. Senile Psychosis
    C. Psychosis with Cerebral Arteriosclerosis
    D. Huntington's Chorea   (20:200)

366. The most important thing to keep in mind while working with a patient with an organic brain syndrome is

    A. his previous level of education
    B. a history of convulsions
    C. the quality of his sensorium
    D. a history of poor nutritional intake   (20:180–81)

367. A mental illness arising from a gunshot wound in the head would be characterized as a/an

    A. psychoneurosis
    B. organic disorder
    C. functional disorder
    D. severe psychogenic disorder   (20:264)

368. A nurse checking to see if a client is correctly oriented should know orientation to

    A. place is the first sphere to go
    B. person is the first sphere to go
    C. time is the last sphere to go
    D. person is the last sphere to go   (20:180–81)

369. Alzheimer's disease and Pick's disease are usually grouped together because both are

    A. due to cerebral arteriosclerosis
    B. presenile psychoses
    C. senile psychoses
    D. due to a vitamin B deficiency   (20:192–95)

370. Epidemiologically, Pick's disease differs from Alzheimer's disease in that Pick's disease

    A. tends to be diagnosed at a slightly earlier age than Alzheimer's
    B. is twice as common in women as in men
    C. might have an hereditary factor
    D. all of the above   (20:192–95)

371. A differential diagnosis between Alzheimer's disease and Pick's disease is extremely difficult. Which of the following symptoms are more common in Pick's disease?

    A. convulsions, facial paresis, and muscular rigidity
    B. aphasic disturbances
    C. indifference and underactivity
    D. motor impulsiveness and aggression
    (20:194–95)

372. Because of the clinical similarities of Alzheimer's disease and Pick's disease, many clinicians feel that a clinical differentiation can be made only on

    A. extensive blood chemistries
    B. post-mortem examination of the brain
    C. thorough prenatal history
    D. none of the above
    (20:194)

373. Which of the following activities would be most important to an elderly client with a diagnosis of organic brain syndrome?

    A. watching television
    B. taking a nap
    C. attending occupational therapy
    D. attending movies
    (21:208)

374. Confabulation is the term used to describe

    A. a state of disordered orientation
    B. the filling in of memory gaps with made-up stories
    C. the quality of being circumstantial; minuteness of detail
    D. a persistent repetitiveness in speech
    (20:120)

375. One of the prime symptomatic differences between senile dementia and cerebral arteriosclerosis is that in cerebral arteriosclerosis, there can occur

    A. a gradual shift in behavioral patterns
    B. a sudden attack of confusion
    C. an easy mental fatigability
    D. all of the above
    (20:198)

376. Cerebral arteriosclerosis accounts for what percentage of first admissions to state psychiatric hospitals?

    A. 10%
    B. 20%
    C. 30%
    D. 40%
    (21:204)

377. The presenting picture of a client with psychosis due to cerebral arteriosclerosis is most like that of a client with

    A. schizophrenia
    B. Alzheimer's disease
    C. tertiary syphilis
    D. depression
    (20:201)

378. Prodromal symptoms of arteriosclerosis include

    A. fatigue and headache
    B. decreased capacity for prolonged concentration
    C. drowsiness in the late afternoon or evening
    D. all of the above
    (20:198)

379. Treatment for the individual with cerebral arteriosclerosis includes all of the following *except*

    A. mild hydrotherapy
    B. a diet devoid of alcohol
    C. a high cholesterol diet
    D. a low fat diet
    (20:201)

380. The elderly client with cerebral arteriosclerosis may relieve associated delirium by increasing his consumption of

    A. water
    B. coffee
    C. orange juice
    D. bananas
    (21:205)

381. Mr. Fox, age 69, is diagnosed with psychosis with cerebral arteriosclerosis. He has been in the hospital for two weeks. When asked by Mr. Tompkins, the nurse, about what he had done the night before, Mr. Fox replied, "Oh,

I went to the races and then for a couple of beers." Mr. Fox is not allowed out of the hospital. This is an example of

A. denial
B. confabulation
C. ideas of grandeur
D. distractibility   (21:205)

382. In making a differential diagnosis between Acute Organic Brain syndrome with delirious state, and schizophrenia, the former would include

    a. fearfulness, clouding of consciousness with bewilderment, and restlessness
    b. confusion, disorientation, and impairment in thinking
    c. clear sensorium and the ability to retain and recall past events
    d. no memory deficits

A. a only
B. a and b
C. a and c
D. c and d   (20:180–81)

Questions 383 to 387

Mr. Simon, an 82-year-old gentleman, has recently been admitted to a psychiatric hospital. He is irritable, forgetful, and often rather childish in his actions. At times, he misidentifies people on the ward and feels that he is being persecuted.

383. The most therapeutic approach by the nurse toward Mr. Simon would be to

A. feel sorry for him because he has grown old
B. feel sympathy for him because he can't always help himself
C. feel genuine interest in his well-being
D. feel that she must always be patient with him   (21:206)

384. A calendar should be put in a prominent place on the ward since aged persons are often

A. apathetic
B. delusional
C. insecure
D. disoriented   (21:208)

385. Mr. Simon walks up to the nurse and says, "Please let me out. I have to go to work now. The store opens at eight o'clock." The most appropriate response by the nurse would be

A. "Today is a holiday. The store is closed."
B. "Don't worry about the store. Someone else is taking care of it."
C. "You used to own a store, didn't you? Tell me about it."
D. "You don't own a store anymore. Let's go into the day room."   (21:208)

386. In planning Mr. Simon's care, the nurse should be most concerned with

A. helping him to lead a very active life on the unit
B. making sure that he gets the proper amount of rest
C. teaching him good personal hygiene
D. helping him to feel that he is important   (21:208)

387. Mr. Simon has not been eating well since he was admitted. He repeatedly says that no one cares. The most appropriate initial response by the nurse would be to

A. serve small portions of the food in an attractive way
B. ask Mr. Simon which foods he especially likes
C. comment, "I like you. Please eat the food for me."
D. comment, "I'll sit here with you if you'll eat your food."   (21:208)

388. Korsakoff's syndrome is caused by a deficiency in

A. vitamin B
B. vitamin A
C. vitamin C
D. vitamin E   (20:213)

389. An organic psychiatric disorder which must be inherited is

    A. syphilis
    B. Huntington's Chorea
    C. Sydenham's disease
    D. Alzheimer's disease   (20:301–02)

390. A serious but temporary condition common to patients who have undergone open heart surgery is

    A. postoperative psychosis
    B. episodic attacks of hyperventilation or auras
    C. gross disorientation
    D. all of the above   (20:202)

391. Paroxysmal attacks involving paralysis of voluntary movements and postural collapse of the whole body due to emotional excitement are best described as

    A. cataplexy
    B. narcolepsy
    C. epilepsy
    D. apoplexy   (20:253)

392. Sydenham's Chorea (St. Vitus Dance) is thought to be associated with

    A. vitamin B deficiency
    B. streptococcal infection
    C. alcohol
    D. dominant mutation   (20:238)

393. Lupus erythematosus disseminata is most frequently observed in

    A. female adolescents
    B. male adolescents
    C. female children
    D. male adults   (20:303)

394. Induced hypoglycemic states are more frequent in

    A. female nurses
    B. pharmacists
    C. medical students
    D. teen-agers   (20:280)

Questions 395 to 396

Mrs. Roy is a 70-year-old woman who has been admitted to the hospital with a diagnosis of senile psychosis.

395. The behavior exhibited by Mrs. Roy is most likely to have been influenced by

    A. the amount of her brain tissue that has been affected
    B. the amount of cholesterol she consumed throughout her life
    C. her particular premorbid personality traits
    D. the amount of alcohol she consumed in the last 20 years   (20:184)

396. Mrs. Roy complains to the nurse that the food "is no good." The most likely explanation for this is that Mrs. Roy

    A. thinks that she is being poisoned
    B. is trying to get attention
    C. has suffered an approximate 50% loss in taste buds
    D. is unable to see what she is eating   (20:184)

397. Diagnosis of senile dementia is most often made between the ages of

    A. 40 to 45 years
    B. 50 to 55 years
    C. 55 to 60 years
    D. 65 to 70 years   (20:185)

398. All of the following characteristics are frequently found in the history of the person who develops senile dementia *except*

    A. rigid and static habits
    B. an abrupt shift in behavioral patterns
    C. constricted life style
    D. long term feelings of insecurity   (20:184–85)

399. In a client with a history of syphilis, it is most important to

    A. obtain a blood test
    B. begin treatment with penicillin

C. obtain cerebrospinal fluid tests
D. check the pupil response   (21:199)

400. The first physical complaint of general paresis is usually that of

A. headaches
B. incontinence
C. slurred speech
D. tremors   (21:200)

401. Which of the following statements about general paresis is true?

A. 25% of the patients are male
B. 75% of the patients are female
C. 75% of the patients are male
D. 50% of the patients are male   (21:199)

402. The most common age for the diagnosis of general paresis is

A. 20 years
B. 25 years
C. 40 years
D. 65 years   (21:199)

403. The chronic brain syndrome or occlusive disease that affects the nutrient vessels of the brain, heart or kidney by progressively choking off the flow of blood is

a. atherosclerosis
b. arteriosclerosis
c. Pick's disease
d. Alzheimer's disease

A. a only
B. a and b
C. c only
D. c and d   (20:196)

404. One might find all of the following in a patient with an organic brain disorder of neurosyphilis *except*

A. negative colloidal gold curve in spinal fluid
B. positive blood and spinal Wasserman tests
C. pupillary changes
D. inability to calculate   (20:228)

405. Port-wine urine is a symptom of

A. porphyria
B. phenylketonuria
C. Wernicke's syndrome
D. hepatolenticular degeneration   (20:285)

406. What factor has been most influential in producing the greatest decrease in the number of cases of general paresis?

A. better community case finding
B. better hygienic conditions
C. the development of thorazine therapy
D. improved antileutic therapy   (20:223)

407. In the Face-Hand Test, a diagnostic test for brain damage, the examiner might expect the client to perform

A. better with his eyes opened than with his eyes closed
B. better with his eyes closed than with his eyes opened
C. the same with his eyes opened as with them closed
D. better if the client is also depressed   (6:III:830)

408. In the Face-Hand Test, exosomethesia refers to the client's reporting the touch to a hand as being

A. a touch to the cheek
B. a touch to the examiner's hand
C. not felt
D. outside himself in space   (6:III:829)

Chapter III: Answers and Explanations

1. **D.** Neurosis is an emotional maladaption characterized chiefly by anxiety arising from some unresolved unconscious conflicts. This anxiety is either felt directly or controlled by various psychological mechanisms to produce other subjectively distressing symptoms.

2. **D.** In neurosis, the patient is aware that there is a disturbance with his mental functioning. There is no gross distortion of external reality and the symptoms are ego alien. He finds the symptoms to be strange, undesirable, unwanted or upsetting.

3. **A.** Neurotic symptoms are strange, undesirable, unwanted, irritating or upsetting. They are ego alien.

4. **C.** The hypochondriacal type occupies a borderline position between the neuroses and psychoses. Hypochondriacal neurosis is the result of a severe regression.

5. **A.** In psychoneurotic disorders, the ego is called upon to exert a continuous and unusual amount of effort in the control of forbidden impulses, either because of the exceptional strength of such impulses, or because of their especially unacceptable nature. The personality is in a state of chronic fatigue and does not have sufficient reserve energy to deal with many environmental stresses, even if these are mild.

6. **C.** Karen Horney developed this theory in her book, *Neurosis and Human Growth*.

7. **A.** Obsessional thoughts are persistent, unwanted ideas and impulses that cannot be eliminated by logic or reasoning.

8. **D.** Severe regression is the fundamental mechanism. Like the infant, the hypochondriac is quite aware of figures in his environment, but he is not able to give to them emotionally. A large part of the libido has been withdrawn from environmental figures and reinvested in various parts of his own body.

9. **A.** The patient's anxiety becomes detached from a specific idea, object, or situation in his daily life and is displaced to some situation in the form of a specific neurotic fear. The fear that he experiences in the presence of the phobic object or experience is the displaced fear of some anxiety-producing component within his own personality. The phobic object or experience symbolizes or represents the incident arousing affects which must be prevented from coming to the surface.

10. **D.** Hysterical neurosis, conversion type, unlike the psychophysiologic disorders is not usually life-threatening. The voluntary and sensory systems are the ones normally involved in the symptomatology.

11. **C.** Since there is a stigma attached to psychological problems in America, many seem to develop physiological problems which they focus on. People allay anxiety by somaticizing despite the absence of physiologic causative factors other than those experienced with anxiety.

12. **B.** Examination of the client usually fails to reveal a responsible organic basis for the production of the symptom.

13. **C.** During W.W. I, there were 60,000 cases of "Disordered Action of the Heart" in the British Army. Internists were unaware that they were dealing with anxiety.

14. **B.** As long as there is a recognition of the nonsensical quality of the symptom and an attempt to resist the symptom, it is a true obsessional neurosis.

15. **C.** It is characteristic of obsessive behavior that guilty fear is always somewhat stronger and it represses defiant rage.

16. **E.** Rank saw this separation as the basic pattern for all separations with its physiological symptoms as a model for anxiety.

17. **C.** Freud originally viewed repressed instinctual or innate drives (unconscious) to be central to the causation of anxiety.

18. **D.** Sullivan sees anxiety as an interpersonal concept rather than as instinctual.

19. **B.** Hostility is anticipated by others during interaction and sensed by the anxious person himself. Anxiety is seen as related to a fear of disruption of one's interpersonal relationships.

20. **A.** Anxiety is connected with anticipated fear of disapproval, withdrawal of love, disruption of interpersonal relationships, isolation, or separation.

21. **C.** Developmentally, the mastery of coordination enables the obsessive to grandiosely overestimate the might of his hands and feet.

22. **D.** Secondary gains are environmental and provide a channel through which culture shapes symptoms.

23. **A.** Class-linked behaviors reflect the relative priorities of defense mechanisms determined by different developmental experiences, that is, educational as well as innate capacities and knowledge and skills acquired by the person during development.

24. **B.** In apparent contradiction to not showing concern about a particular symptom in the patient's presence, the nurse should evaluate every symptom carefully for its medical or psychological significance.

25. **D.** In a conversion reaction, anxiety is converted into functional symptoms in organs or parts of the body innervated by the sensorimotor nervous system. The conversion symptoms serve to prevent or lessen any conscious, felt anxiety (la belle indifference) and usually symbolize the underlying mental conflict that is productive of anxiety.

26. **A.** Freud explained the hysterical symptoms as caused by a conflict between the superego and some wish that, because of its consciously objectionable nature, is repressed. This repression is not entirely successful, and the wish obtains disguised expression by its "conversion" into the symptom. The nature and localization of this symptom symbolize the repressed wish.

27. **D.** The conversion mechanism yields a primary or neurotic gain through its anxiety-defense function. The concept is that mental states, both normal and pathological, develop defensively in largely unconscious attempts to cope with or to resolve unconscious conflicts.

28. **C.** In the obsessive-compulsive reaction, the patient's anxiety is automatically controlled by associating it with persistently repetitive thoughts and acts.

29. **C.** The patient recognizes that his unwanted thoughts and ritualistic acts are unreasonable, but he is unable to control them.

30. **D.** The function of compulsive acts is to allay or bind anxiety. If the patient is prevented from carrying out his compulsive ritual, overt anxiety appears. The loss of control (slapping the nurse) was most likely due to the intolerable anxiety.

31. **B.** It is important for the nurse to recognize her own feelings about aggressive behavior and to help the patient set limits on unacceptable aggressive behavior. More appropriate ways of expressing aggression may be developed as the patient discusses his thoughts and feelings with the nurse.

32. **D.** In the obsessive-compulsive reaction, anxiety is controlled by associating it with persistently repetitive thoughts and acts. Ritualistic activities are performed in an effort to dispel or counteract the thoughts.

33. **B.** When another member of the health team is the primary therapist, the nurse plays a collaborative role. She provides a psychotherapeutic milieu for the patient and supplements the primary therapist's data collection and assessment by sharing observations and facts.

34. **B.** The primary, unconscious purpose of the conversion reaction is to provide relief from the distressing anxiety produced by the emotional situation responsible for the occurrence of the physical symptom. The symptoms usually are those of the voluntary nervous system.

35. **C.** The learning theory model is that of extinction of traumatic avoidance reactions. These reactions are difficult to extinguish under conditions where one is free to avoid or escape the noxious stimulus.

36. **B.** In a neurotic depression, the client ordinarily becomes increasingly low-spirited as the day progresses.

37. **A.** The higher economic and social classes seek psychiatric treatment for psychoneurotic disorders. The middle class usually seeks medical treatment.

38. **A.** The patient consciously recognizes that no actual danger exists but cannot control the overwhelming feeling of dread.

39. **C.** The three forms are (1) persistent recurrence of an unwelcome thought, (2) a morbid and often irresistible urge to perform a certain repetitive, stereotyped act and (3) an obsessively recurring thought accompanied by a compulsion to perform a repetitive act.

40. **C.** She should explain that the medication is to diminish anxiousness and not to treat any physical disorder.

41. **D.** The psychoneurotic patient is often skillful in his attempts to draw the nurse into a social relationship and this may undermine subsequent therapeutic intervention by the nurse.

42. **E.** The rituals indicate the utilization of undoing.

43. **D.** Certain strivings and emotions are unconsciously transferred from one object, activity, or situation to another.

44. **A.** The internal conflict between the good and bad parts of the introjected object results in guilt and self reproach.

45. **B.** Certain aspects of activities of the personality escape from the control of the individual.

46. **C.** Psychological material is converted into physical manifestations.

47. **A.** It is a fictionalized account of a multiple personality, a severe dissociative reaction.

48. **B.** The physical symptom observed is symbolic of the underlying conflict which produced the disability to prevent or relieve anxiety.

49. **B.** The nurse must remain calm when dealing with a patient with an acute anxiety attack, for if the patient sees alarm in the nurse, he promptly assumes that his fears of severe mental or physical disease are confirmed by her attitude.

50. **C.** The value of "rest" is doubtful for many anxious patients. Many patients are more comfortable when they are busy. Some anxious patients feel worse when they are away from their homes.

51. **A.** The severely compulsive client usually has become socially isolated, for his interests have narrowed to himself and his time-consuming compulsive acts. The nurse attempts to substitute interest in people in place of the patient's interest in his compulsive acts.

52. **D.** The nurse does not challenge or infer doubt of the patient's physical complaints but avoids demonstrating serious concern of them. Constant reassurance is undesirable because it stimulates new symptoms and greater fear. Repeated physical examinations tend to emphasize organic causes.

53. **B.** A phobia is believed to arise through a process of displacing an internal (unconscious) conflict to an external object symbolically related to the conflict.

54. **B.** Hysterical symptoms are often removed or diminished by strong suggestion through hypnosis or barbiturate interviews. Suggestive methods should be accompanied by psychotherapy.

55. **C.** Acro comes from the Greek word *akrow* or promontory. Acrophobia is a pathological dread of high places.

56. **E.** Scoto is from Greek meaning "darkness." Scotophobia is an abnormal fear of darkness.

57. **H.** Myso comes from the Greek *mysos*, meaning filth. Mysophobia means fear of dirt or filth.

58. **G.** Claustro comes from the Latin word *claustrum* meaning enclosure; thus, claustrophobia means a dread of closed or narrow places.

59. **A.** *Aqua* is the Latin word for water. Aquaphobia is the morbid fear of water.

60. **F.** *Myth* is a Greek word meaning legendary story. Mythophobia is the dread of stating something that is not absolutely accurate.

61. **D.** *Agora* is a Greek word meaning marketplace or place for a political assembly. Agoraphobia is a morbid fear of being in an open space.

62. **B.** *Pyro* is the Greek combination form for fire. Pyrophobia is a dread of fire.

63. **J.** *Arachnes* is the Greek word meaning spider or spider's web. Arachnephobia means a morbid fear of spiders.

64. **I.** *Mono* is from Greek meaning alone or single. Monophobia is the fear of being alone.

65. **A.** The Ganser syndrome is a rare type of hysterical dissociative reaction which occurs in prisoners awaiting trial. The patient has confusion, memory loss, disorientation and, at times, hallucinations.

66. **B.** The obsessive patient has no urge for his obsession to be carried out, but a dread that it will occur. For example, the patient with an obsessive fear of suicide, has no urge to commit suicide but has a persistent fear that he may do so.

67. **B.** Anxiety is the basic symptom in psychoneurosis, although in the conversion reaction, one notes a peculiar calm or indifference known as la belle indifference.

68. **D.** During World War I, it was noted that enlisted men who came from lower socioeconomic groups had a high rate of conversion reaction, whereas, the officers suffered from anxiety reactions. In W.W. II, the enlisted men, who were recruited from the middle class had psychosomatic complaints rather than conversion symptoms.

69. **C.** The clinical picture in psychoneurosis is generally a mixed one. Psychoneurotic symptoms can also occur in psychoses, psychosomatic disturbances, and personality disorders.

70. **D.** How the question is phrased is important. The nurse's response invites validation of the feelings communicated by the patient.

71. **C.** If the nurse attacks the defense of the patient, the patient will feel more anxious. Peplau says that by permitting the patient's mechanisms to operate, possibly his feelings of security will become strong enough that he will feel safe to doubt what he is doing.

72. **A.** The handwashing ritual is an adaptation to reduce or avoid the anxiety.

73. **C.** The mechanism is undoing. The anxiety is temporarily alleviated by the compulsive washing, with its symbolic significance.

74. **A.** Thoughts that persistently thrust themselves into consciousness against the conscious desire of the patient are known as obsessions. Obsessive thoughts are unwanted.

75. **C.** Anxiety states rank highest in the number of neurotic problems encountered in outpatient psychiatric work.

76. **C.** The patient is given free reign to express his feelings and to choose his activities.

77. **D.** Resolving these conflicts is crucial, because the effectiveness of milieu therapy can be destroyed by competitiveness, hostility and misunderstandings between staff members and many patients are upset by them.

78. **C.** The manifestations of anxiety are both somatic and experiential. The somatic are the result of autonomic nervous system discharges; the experiential ones consist of the patient's conscious awareness of the somatic processes.

79. **D.** The nurse can lower the level of the patient's anxiety by her presence. An anxious patient should not be isolated from human contact.

80. **A.** Anxiety is engendered by deep, unconscious, unrecognized conflict and displaced into observable symptoms.

81. **B.** Amnesia is a dissociative experience in which the person's recollection is lost or split off from conscious recall. It may be functional or organic in origin.

82. **B.** In a conversion reaction, anxiety, instead of being consciously experienced, is "converted" into functional symptoms in organs or parts of the body innervated by the sensorimotor nervous system.

83. **D.** Phobias are reported to be twice as common among women as among men.

84. **B.** These individuals have weak superegos. If ego ideals exist, they are directed to narcissistic goals and the control of others for immediate pleasures.

85. **D.** Antisocial personalities are usually callous and given to immediate pleasures.

86. **D.** The future antisocial personality is often that of an unwanted child or one whose parental relationship has terminated in desertion or divorce. The patient's mother has frequently had a very unhappy childhood. The adolescent is usually antagonistic and resistant to the ideals and mores of his family.

87. **B.** Moral and ethical blunting and inconsistencies of behavior are constantly demonstrated. Although plausible and talkative, he is absolutely unreliable.

88. **D.** Concurrent with the establishment of a warm accepting environment, it is essential that a sense of authority be consistently and firmly maintained. Infractions of behavior should be treated with loss of privileges and their reinstitution on improved behavior.

89. **C.** Research studies indicate a limited degree of success in working with persons with antisocial personality disorders. The prognosis, of course, is dependent on many individual variables. Ideally, the nurse would wish to explore with the parents, their thoughts and concerns regarding Doris' future.

90. **D.** Although the people on skid row have formerly been thought of as comprising the alcoholic population, these individuals are not all alcoholic and make up only five percent of alcoholics.

91. **C.** Fifty percent of alcoholics attended or graduated from college. Forty-five percent are employed at a professional or managerial level. Thirteen percent received only grammar school education and thirty-seven percent are high school graduates. Five percent are unemployed and twenty-five percent are white collar workers.

92. **A.** Bulimia is morbidly increased hunger. Polyphagia is pathological overeating.

93. **B.** Neurotic alcoholism refers to the type of excessive drinking that is based on some unconscious motivation and serves as a means for maintaining equilibrium for the person. In this instance, there would be relief of anxiety.

94. **A.** Families of alcoholics tend to follow a pattern in their attempts to handle the problem. Initially, the efforts take the form of denial as they pretend that all is normal.

95. **B.** Intoxication depends upon the amount of alcohol in the blood stream. A concentration of 0.10 to 0.20 percent in the blood indicates intoxification whereas 0.50 to 0.90 percent is in the fatal range.

96. **C.** Physical restraints may frighten the client and he can exhaust himself struggling against them. Bed rails should not be used as the client often attempts to climb over them.

97. **B.** It is estimated that ten million American families deal with this problem daily. These families have the potential for becoming disorganized as evidenced by the higher rate of divorce and separation among alcoholics.

98. **D.** The alcohol addict can obtain alcohol legally; the narcotic addict cannot. Alcohol tends to release aggression whereas narcotics inhibit it. The drug addict functions well as long as he obtains enough drugs to ward off his abstinence syndrome. The chronically intoxicated alcoholic cannot function normally as long as he maintains his intoxicating intake of alcohol.

99. **B.** Before taking the initiative, the nurse explains the therapeutic regime to the patient.

100. **D.** Alcohol taken in moderation stimulates the flow of digestive juices and thereby aids digestion.

101. **D.** The one characteristic common to all alcoholics is that they drink too much. The idea of an alcoholic personality is no longer accepted.

102. **C.** There is considerable agreement that persons manifesting sexual deviations have been arrested in their psychosexual development at some earlier level of emotional growth.

103. **B.** A voyeur is a person with a compulsive interest in watching or looking at others, particularly at genitals.

104. **B.** The sociopath would probably observe the power structure in an attempt to vie for leadership and control as well as to play staff and patients against one another.

105. **B.** Antisocial behavior is characterized by an inability to love and feel affection as well as the tendency to act on impulse. It is largely manipulative in nature.

106. **D.** Nurses need to set limits on behaviors which violate basic rules of health and safety.

107. **C.** Alcoholics have deep inner feelings of inferiority, insecurity, fear of rejection, and anxiety.

108. **A.** Feelings of anxiety and guilt cause the alcoholic to become completely dependent upon alcohol to ease the discomfort of threatening influences.

109. **C.** Well-lit rooms help to reduce the fears and illusory experiences of the delirious alcoholic. The nurse should approach quietly and speak gently to these patients.

110. **A.** Members of Alanon endeavor to learn about alcoholism in an effort to understand better the effects of their relationships with the alcoholic partners.

111. **G.** These persons fail in their emotional, economic, occupational, and social adjustment.

112. **F.** Schizoid persons avoid close relationships with others, are unable to express hostility, and manifest autistic thinking.

113. **A.** Cyclothymic behavior is superficial with emotional reaching out to the environment.

114. **B.** Paranoid persons are extremely sensitive in interpersonal relations and have a tendency to utilize projection.

115. **C.** Even under minor stress, these individuals react with excitability which is ineffective. One never knows whether they are friend or foe.

116. **D.** These individuals deal with aggressive feelings through behavior that is dependent, passive or outwardly hostile.

117. **E.** These individuals demonstrate chronic, excessive concern with adherence to standards of conscience or of conformity.

118. **D.** The prognosis becomes poor when the person has been addicted early in life, has a low educational level, and a short employment history.

119. **D.** Inappropriate identification with opposite-sexed parents, role reversal of parents and easier access to sexual gratification from one's own sex during adolescence are considered factors in the causation of homosexuality.

120. **C.** This approach has emotional appeal and a somewhat salesmanship quality.

121. **D.** Any two of these factors are sufficient to support an addiction. Other factors are: the properties of the chemical, social support of other users, and the lack of job skills or schooling.

122. **A.** Special inpatient facilities are probably always needed, although not necessarily a hospital. Usually, the institution has been correctional in nature. Institutions in existence, have reported successful treatment of severe cases in three to five years.

123 **B.** Cleckley's *The Mask of Sanity* and Aichhorn's *The Wayward Youth* are both accounts of psychotherapy with sociopathic clients.

124. **D.** The team approach enables the hostility and incessant demands to be shared rather than focused on the therapist alone.

125. **C.** All persons with suicidal ideation have an intense underlying sense of deprivation of affection and love, and a deep sense of personal rejection. His suicidal attempt may or may not be related to his homosexuality. The data is insufficient to make an interpretation.

126. **D.** Synanon is an organization of former addicts for addicts who volunteer to eliminate their habit. The addict withdraws from his habit without the support of any drugs and without the supervision of a physician.

127. **D.** Each member faces a totally different group each session so that a member cannot protect another member from revealing painful material.

128. **D.** Chafetz reports the antipathy and lack of understanding of the therapists to be the greatest drawback.

129. **A.** There are two federal hospitals for the treatment of drug addiction, one in Lexington, Kentucky, the other in Fort Worth, Texas.

130. **C.** Approximately fifty percent of these deaths occurred in the young, and the same percentage was due to overdosage. These high rates reflect the new patterns of narcotic use as well as the highly variable dosages available in supplies provided through the illicit market. These statistics are from a study of New York City.

131. **C.** According to Yahraes, there needs to be a psychologically maladjusted individual, an available drug, and a mechanism for bringing them together.

132. **B.** Ordinarily, the addict is introduced to drugs by his associates.

133. **D.** Withdrawal symptoms may include tremors, excessive perspiration, nausea, vomiting, anorexia, restlessness, hallucinations, convulsions and delirium tremens.

134. **B.** Threatening behavior of the manipulative patient is illustrated in this example.

135. **A.** Asking for clarification, elaboration and details of the situation implies a concern for the client.

136. **C.** The fetishist is unable to love a real person but becomes attached to some material object having a feminine association. Contact with this object leads to orgasm.

137. **C.** There is faulty superego control; the pathology is directed against others and does not cause guilt, anxiety or depression. The pathology is expressed by their behavior rather than psychotic, somatic or neurotic symptoms.

138. **D.** The key figures with whom Joseph identified have standards or values which are at variance with the general society.

139. **B.** Shadows cast by bright corridor lights upon the walls and ceilings of a dimly lit or darkened room may be stimuli which induce illusions of animals, bugs, or other disturbing objects.

140. **A.** Bed rest is desirable and symptomatic treatment until the severe pain subsides.

141. **A.** This position will prevent the occurrence of foot drop.

142. **D.** One of the fundamental ideas of A. A. is that an alcoholic can receive the most effective help from those who have experienced the same difficulty and thus gain true acceptance.

143. **A.** The patient with Korsakoff's psychosis is usually disoriented as to that which is beyond immediate observation and dependent on memory.

144. **D.** The therapeutic handling of manipulative behavior depends upon the firm, consistent setting of limits on behavior.

145. **D.** Heroin produces constriction of the pupils.

146. **A.** Generally, opiate and barbiturate dependence seems to originate in socially deprived areas.

147. **D.** The nurse's emotional reaction to the manipulative behavior is the first consideration. As control of one's feelings is accomplished, the nurse can identify and acknowledge the uncomfortable feelings. The nurse needs to have her own feelings under control to be therapeutic. Then it is necessary to understand the meaning of the behavior and to assess how the patient understands what he does. Validation of the meaning of the behavior comes from staff discussion. Staff, to be therapeutic, need to present a unified approach to the manipulative behavior.

148. **A.** Encouraging the verbal expression of feelings helps to teach new behavior to the client.

149. **B.** Severe addiction to morphine, over a long period of time, produces no appreciable damage to bodily tissue. Physical addiction to marihuana does not occur. It affects the emotions, social, academic and vocational performance in a deleterious way.

150. **B.** Since amphetamines are appetite suppressors, he is usually malnourished.

151. **C.** Persons who misuse amphetamines occasionally develop paranoid psychotic states in which they fear people are trying to rob and kill them.

152. **C.** Drug abuse is common in the professions. Among occupational groups, physicians, pharmacists, and nurses have a high rate.

153. **C.** Habitual drinkers do, in a minority of cases, develop some tolerance to alcohol. A portion of what passes for tolerance among habitual heavy drinkers is actually psychological tolerance. Physiologic tolerance for morphine is usual.

154. **B.** Chafetz reports that the nurse needs a chance to examine her own feelings and reactions to alcoholic patients.

155. **B.** The report of the Committee on Alcoholism of the Council on Mental Health of the American Medical Association was published in 1956.

156. **C.** In 1944, the National Committee on Alcoholism and the Yale Plan Clinic in New Haven were established.

157. **C.** The most important aspect of management of delirium tremens is to make certain that the client is well hydrated and to correct any electrolyte imbalance.

158. **C.** Delirium tremens ends fatally in about fifteen percent of untreated cases.

159. **B.** Observation has indicated that there are a number of alternative courses for alcoholism to take. The view that all alcoholic persons if untreated, will show a progressive downhill course, is incorrect.

160. **A.** Such determination and loyalty are not characteristic of the antisocial personality.

161. **D.** These drinking practices tend to maximize the desired effects of alcohol and minimize the adverse effects.

162. **B.** Addicts who have used opiates for as long as fifty years have shown no evidence of mental deterioration.

163. **D.** Symptoms of withdrawal from morphine-like narcotics include all of those listed as well as increased respiratory rate, profuse sweating, mydriasis, and rhinorrhea.

164. **B.** Amphetamine psychosis is characterized by ideas of reference and delusions of persecution.

165. **B.** These drugs are psychodelic and produce heightened awareness.

166. **D.** Three aspects of psychological changes include: (1) concern with alcohol, (2) denial, and (3) self-loathing.

167. **B.** In the mild abstinence syndrome, symptoms resemble those of a common cold or an allergic reaction.

168. **C.** Pedophilics are males with a sexual preference for girls and/or boys under the age of 16. They usually have a heterosexual orientation and frequently are married.

169. **D.** Transvestites prefer women as sexual partners and in fantasies of sex. They do not appear effeminate.

170. **C.** Although there is some overlap among the various sexual variants, the majority of cases fit into one category. Males who receive emotional and sexual gratification by dressing as women are called transvestites.

171. **C.** As a result of this committee's report to Parliament and subsequent changes in the laws, all sexual activity between consenting adults in private is legal in Great Britain.

172. **D.** Ambition and physical energy are lessened; lethargy is produced, and the individual pays less attention to work.

173. **B.** The loss of one's job presents a severe threat to one's self-confidence and self-esteem. This is particularly true for the man who is nearing the retirement age.

174. **C.** Important to the recovery process is the nurse's need to deal with the client's fear since his illness threatens his total integrity as well as his sense of personal adequacy and worth to others. The nurse needs to help the client find adequate situational support and also to use the problem solving approach in order to resolve this difficulty.

175. **C.** Since the time of Hippocrates, it has been known that a relationship exists between emotional arousal and the precipitation of an asthmatic attack. Although there is usually a constitutional predisposition for asthma, emotional factors, such as an unusually strong maternal dependency, affect the client.

176. **B.** Persisting strong infantile longings to be loved and cared for are often compensated for by aggressive ambitious, and driving personality characteristics.

177. **D.** Pseudocyesis (false pregnancy) is influenced both by the wish for and fear of pregnancy. Certain immature women present themselves with many of the signs of pregnancy including cessation of menses, distention of the abdomen, changes in the breasts and increase in weight.

178. **B.** Although emotional conflict is a causative factor, there is no symbolic meaning in the physical findings of psychosomatic disorders. The symptoms are not expressive of anything and have no adaptive values. In contrast to the psychoneurotic, the person with a psychophysiologic disorder may not be aware of his disease for a considerable time. Since there is no adaptive value, there can be no primary gain.

179. **C.** Frequently there is an undercurrent deeply repressed, of a need for mother or a fear of estrangement from mother or a mother substitute. The asthmatic attacks have been viewed as symbolic cries for mother.

180. **D.** Mr. Greene is unconsciously rejecting that which is consciously intolerable. His overdependency on his wife is not a healthy way of dealing with the reality of his colostomy.

181. **D.** Aortic stenosis and mitral insufficiency can induce psychotic reactions. Hepatic disorders can cause hallucinations in the absence of anxiety. Renal insufficiency may produce apathy, depression, confusion, and agitation. Hyperthyroid patients can develop psychoses.

182. **B.** With a psychophysiologic disorder, a pathological emotional state may precipitate or aggravate the illness while a more satisfactory psychological state may facilitate the healing process.

183. **C.** The evidence for the significance of personality "types" in the production of somatic illness is very weak.

184. **C.** The psychophysiologic disorders involve suppressed or repressed emotions which gain expression through body organs and organ systems.

185. **C.** Distracting them from arguing is the goal. To directly handle and control the arguing at the bedside would not be an easy task. To tell the children that they should or should not argue would probably set up feelings in the father that his children were bad or that he was not exercising adequate control.

186. **B.** The best approach would be to try to take the children aside at some point during the visit so that they can discuss with the nurse their feelings about what it is like to have their father in the hospital. Once a rapport has been established, the nurse would attempt to discuss the family dynamics with all of the members present.

187. **D.** The beginning therapeutic task for the nurse would be to encourage the client to talk. An important issue for him would be to talk about his feelings.

188. **D.** A peptic ulcer may be interpreted as the inappropriate perpetuation of organic reactions adaptive to, or protective against, some stress in the client's life.

189. **D.** The nurse utilizes the techniques of restating without attacking or labeling his feelings and thus gives him a chance to explore them. She recognizes that Mr. Gallagher may not be aware of his fear, that he may have dissociated it.

190. **D.** The distinguishing signs are: (1) it occurs mostly in teen-age girls, (2) the reduction in dietary intake is psychically determined, (3) vomiting occurs and is sometimes self-induced, and (4) amenorrhea, constipation, and cachexia are present.

191. **C.** The patient needs attention at mealtime. Sitting with her may help. If the patient is punishing herself by not eating, adding more punishment is not effective.

192. **A.** Inner tension may be partly repressed and suppressed, but the resulting mild-mannered facade covers conflicting attitudes of readiness for aggressive hostility with needs to conform in order to maintain strong dependent attachments, especially to authority figures.

193. **D.** All of the statements given are correct. Although the personality of many hypertensive patients is that of outward serenity and affability, many are neurotic with strong perfectionistic and compulsive tendencies. Although many of the symptoms seem to be of emotional origin, there is a considerable amount of evidence suggesting hereditary factors.

194. **B.** Denial is one of the most frequent adaptive mechanisms used by patients with psychophysiologic cardiovascular disorders.

195. **B.** Nurses can often help a hypertensive patient understand and alleviate his unexpressed anger, but they cannot interpret the high blood pressure as being a substitute for, an expression of, or a defense against the anger, for it is none of these.

196. **A.** Psychoanalytic studies have shown that peptic ulcer patients have a persisting strong infantile wish to be loved and cared for, conflicting with the adult drive for independence.

197. **B.** The drive to be cared for is equated with that to be fed and thus associated with gastric hyperactivity. The intrapsychic conflict when heightened by external circumstances can induce shameful anxiety.

198. **C.** Although at one time peptic ulcers were prevalent in women, they now occur chiefly in men. They are also more frequently seen in those subject to depression and alcoholism and are uncommon in schizophrenics.

199. **D.** Although the ulcer patient and his parents are probably genetically predisposed, there is clear evidence to support the clinical impression that functional gastric symptoms commonly follow worry, business reverses, family quarrels and other emotionally disturbing experiences.

200. **C.** Depression refers both to a symptom and to a group of illnesses that have certain features in common. The psychodynamic mechanisms that are related to the blow to his self-esteem are: identification, the relation of anger to depression, the role of isolation and denial, the evolution of manic states, and the relationship between depression and projective defenses.

201. **A.** Traditionally, depression has been considered an illness of the middle-aged and elderly. Most studies show that depression, unlike the other psychiatric illnesses, is more common in married individuals.

202. **A.** The cognitive signs and symptoms of depression include the patient's distorted view of himself, his world, and his future. The patient views himself as deficient and anticipates making incorrect decisions.

203. **D.** The basic physiological signs of depression include: anorexia, weight loss, constipation, amenorrhea, insomnia and "morning-evening variation in symptoms."

204. **C.** Endogenous depressions are viewed as the expression of a constitutionally determined reaction pattern that is relatively unaffected by external events.

205. **D.** Loss, whether due to separation from or death of a loved one, is the most common cause of depression. Separation of the young child from the mothering figure can produce severe physiological and psychological disturbances.

206. **C.** Object loss, be it death or separation from a loved one, loss of a body part, loss of a job, or loss of a life style, results in either the normal process of mourning or the pathological process of depression.

207. **A.** In order for the loss to be resolved, hypercathexis must take place. That is, the remembering completely and realistically of all the pleasures and disappointments of the lost relationship.

208. **C.** Any important loss is accompanied by pain and despair because of the persistent and insatiable nature of the yearning for the lost object.

209. **A.** If a person completes his grief work, reviews his relationship in both its positive and negative aspects, the ego is freed to invest in a new object or goal.

210. **B.** There are several features that differentiate normal mourning from pathological depression. The grief-stricken individual does not suffer from a diminution of self-esteem, nor is he irrationally guilty.

211. **B.** When an ambivalently loved object is lost, the energy that has been bound up in the loved one is relocated in the ego. The identification with the lost one is equally ambivalently perceived, and mourning takes a pathological turn and becomes depression because the hostile feelings once directed toward the loved one are now being turned against a part of the self.

212. **C.** The initial stage of grief and mourning is denial.

213. **C.** Parents who are experiencing loss, as of a spouse, need assistance in expressing their thoughts and feelings while in the presence of their children as long as they avoid becoming overwrought and hysterical.

214. **C.** A principle therapeutic task for someone who has suffered a loss is that of catharsis. It is essential that the individual be allowed to "talk out" and experience the appropriate emotional reactions, both positive feelings and negative feelings.

215. **C.** Dimunition in self-confidence and self-esteem are cardinal symptoms of depression and not normal grieving.

216. **B.** When a person is unable to work through the normal mourning process, the emotionally charged representation of the lost one remains a permanent part of the self or it becomes introjected. The faults of the lost person become allied with the patient's ego and thus become a punitive superego.

217. **A.** Lindemann studied these Boston families who had been left and thus were suddenly and unexpectedly bereaved. He identified five points which establish the diagnosis of grief.

218. **D.** Any significant loss whether that of a loved one, body part, role, etc. can lead to a process of mourning over the "lost object".

219. **D.** Differentiating features between normal mourning and pathological depression are the diminution of self-esteem and the irrational feelings of guilt in the latter.

220. **A.** Taking the initiative, after an explanation to the patient, indicates that the patient is expected to carry through his therapeutic regime. Ruesch calls this technique, "unagressive directness."

221. **C.** A regular, but not rigid, schedule of activities often relieves the depressed patient of the anxiety he feels about making decisions and his fear of making wrong ones. These fears often freeze him into inactivity and therefore a schedule drawn up by the nurse is necessary to introduce him into ward programs.

222. **B.** It is typical of the psychotically depressed patient to be at his worst in the early morning hours and to experience a slight elevation of mood as the day progresses.

223. **A.** Loss of appetite rather than an increase in appetite is a common symptom of depression. Dry mouth is not a common symptom of depression.

224. **D.** The nurse takes the time to ensure that time is set aside for eating and, if necessary, she stays with the patient.

225. **A.** The manic patient frequently sleeps only three or four hours a night and may lose weight because of overactivity and poor eating.

226. **C.** A manic patient often eats and drinks little, and this, combined with his high energy output, may cause him to lose weight and to become dehydrated. He needs a high caloric intake, often achieved by between-meal snacks.

227. **B.** The nurse should limit the number of fellow patients that the manic patient interacts with. Initially, it is helpful if he carries out his activities alone or in the company of a nurse or aide.

228. **B.** The tempo of a manic patient's hyperactivity is increased by stimulating events in his environment, and conversely, his excitement is decreased by a calming atmosphere.

229. **B.** It is important that the nurse not allow the manic patient to become the center of the group's attention or to lead the group helter-skelter until the group tires of him and rejects him. Low-keyed activities need to be planned by the nurse for the hyperactive patient.

230. **C.** Physical work projects can absorb much of the manic patient's hyperactivity.

231. **C.** Kretschmer described types of body physiques and Jung discussed temperament types. Investigators have linked pyknic types, extroversion, and manic depressive disorders, although the connection has not been considered significant.

232. **C.** The largest number of first attacks of manic depressive psychosis occurs between the ages of twenty and thirty-five.

233. **C.** Competitive activities should be discouraged as they tend to increase his overactivity and overstimulate. Postponement and substitution are two useful diverting techniques that utilize the client's distractibility. Loose supervision helps the client to continue the activity rather than abandon it.

234. **A.** These projects, which require continuous action of the large muscle groups, are better suited to the manic patient than fine, discriminatory work such as knitting and jigsaw puzzles.

235.	**D.** Writing projects can absorb some of the overactivity of manic patients. They do not require fine discriminatory work or competition.

236.	**C.** Flight of ideas is the disturbance of the stream of thought in which the thinking processes appear to run too quickly and as a result, no idea is completed.

237.	**B.** Mrs. Brennan needs help in controlling her hyperactive behavior. Removing her from the day room provides relief from the group stimuli yet, gives her a person to relate to in a quiet environment.

238.	**B.** It is important to recognize that continuous hyperactivity can lead to physical and mental exhaustion.

239.	**B.** Chlorpromazine is a useful adjunct in the early manic stages if the patient is overactive and unmanageable. Because of the hypotensive effect of thorazine, an initial I.M. dose of 25 mg is the most appropriate.

240.	**B.** The manic's behavior is essentially a defense of massive denial against the underlying depression.

241.	**A.** Although both manic patients and patients in catatonic excitement exhibit symptoms of overactivity, the catatonic schizophrenic often expresses the disharmony or inappropriateness between his mood and the ideas expressed.

242.	**A.** The admission rate of manic depressive patients to hospitals in England and Wales exceeds that for the public mental hospitals in the U.S. by 18 times and by 9 times for both public and private mental hospitals.

243.	**D.** The hyperactivity is the mirror image or the denial of a depression. Interpersonal relationships are on a superficial level.

244.	**C.** Just as the depressed patient neglects himself in a self-destructive way, the manic patient neglects himself by compulsive overactivity.

245.	**A.** External stimuli are kept to a minimum. Speaking quietly and slowly helps the client to relax. The client needs what Peplau calls "sustaining thereness" from the nurse.

246.	**A.** Toxic symptoms may occur above serum lithium levels of 1.5 mEq. per liter. Nausea, abdominal cramps, vomiting, diarrhea, thirst, and polyuria are the symptoms indicative of toxicity and suggest the need to reduce the dosage. Toxic symptoms may be reversed by prompt discontinuance of the drug and correction of the abnormalities in the fluid and electrolyte balance.

247.	**D.** Since this is a somatic delusion, the nurse does not try to argue with or convince the patient of the reality. However, she should listen to the complaint and point out the existing reality.

248.	**B.** Although in psychotic depressions there is frequently a regressive move to infantile dependency, the thought disturbances of self-directed rage are expressed in delusions of guilt and shame.

249.	**C.** The patient needs help from the nurse in redirecting her activity. A simple, non-threatening, non-competitive task is frequently successful. The task, however, needs to be one which channels the motor restlessness.

250.	**D.** When the patient states her feelings of depression and worthlessness, the nurse reflects these feeling tones and indicates briefly that she does not share the patient's view of herself. The patient needs to know that these feelings are a part of her illness.

251.	**C.** There is no other mental disorder in which suicidal attempts are as common as in the involutional depression. Therefore, it is essential that the nurse pick up all cues and carefully evaluate the suicidal risk.

252.	**C.** Suicidal risk is considered great when the patient begins to improve, for then he has more energy to carry out the suicidal gesture.

253.	**B.** Depressions that occur at this time of life are caused by emotional traumas. Women undergo many adjustments in their family life, social life, and economic activities in middle-age and these changes, rather than hormonal ones, may play a role in depression.

254.	**C.** This is an example of psychotic ambivalence about his wish to live. The two opposing drives of life and death are present.

255.	**A.** When the nurse assesses the patient as not being in contact with reality, thereby indicating a psychotic state, she assumes control, or sees that someone does, for the person until the psychotic state abates.

256.	**A.** The coexistence of two opposing feelings or emotions toward the same person, object, or goal describes ambivalence. It may be conscious, partly conscious, or one side of the feelings may be conscious.

257.	**C.** Support the client by encouraging her to talk so she can gain insight into the reality of the ambivalent feelings that mothers have from time to time regarding their children. By listening, the nurse can show that she is not afraid to hear these thoughts and feelings. No one can be good or perfect all of the time.

258. **C.** Temper tantrums and accident proneness are evidence of displaced depressive feelings in latency-aged children.

259. **D.** There is a tendency for adolescents to group together to find support in each other and to use drugs or alcohol to escape painful emotions. Sexual activity is frequently attempted to alleviate feelings of loneliness. These are all related to depression. The adolescent may also exhibit symptoms of adult depression such as anorexia, social isolation, and sleeplessness.

260. **D.** Guilt over sexual acting out has been identified as a major factor in suicide attempts by adolescent girls. There seems to be a correlation between youth who commit or attempt suicide, and broken homes. An unstable home life in the five years before the attempt is a factor. Cultural factors increase the suicide rate by producing psychological stresses, by being tolerant towards suicide, and by failing to provide alternative behaviors.

261. **C.** E.S.T. is utilized immediately in these high risk clients since antidepressant medications take two or more weeks to be effective.

262. **D.** In the hospital, there is a positive correlation between a therapeutic milieu and a lower suicide rate. Success in treating suicidal patients is more likely with a therapeutic milieu having easy lines of communication.

263. **C.** The risk of suicide is greatest during weekend leaves from the hospital and shortly after discharge from the hospital.

264. **C.** People tend to commit suicide more often when depression is lifting or after a period in which they have begun to feel better.

265. **C.** Functional mental illness is an illness of an emotional origin in which organic change cannot be demonstrated.

266. **A.** Schizophrenia includes a large group of disorders, usually of psychotic proportion, manifested by characteristic disturbances of thought, mood, and behavior. Thought disturbances are marked by alterations of concept formation that may lead to misinterpretation of reality. Mood changes include ambivalence, constriction, inappropriateness, and loss of empathy with others. Behavior may be withdrawn, regressive, and bizarre.

267. **C.** Bleuler designated as primary symptoms those that he considered were the direct manifestations of a hypothetical somatic morbid process; these included: a peculiar loosening of the associational links in thinking, a morbid ambitendence and ambivalence that dominates the affective life of the patient and a tendency to replace reality by fantasy, a quality that is responsible for the various manifestations of autism.

268. **B.** Bleuler believed that the secondary symptoms were attempts at adaptation to the primary disturbance. They include: delusions explainable by the patient's frustrations and hopes, a part of the hallucinations, the mannerisms, the catatonic muscular symptoms, and a large part of the complicated attitudes that others had called deterioration or dementia.

269. **C.** They are merely convenient ways of describing schizophrenic patients in terms of their predominant symptoms.

270. **D.** Even at present, the etiology of schizophrenia poses important unsolved questions. In a consideration of etiology, the possible factors may conveniently be divided into two groups: organic and psychogenic.

271. **D.** Twin studies have shown a higher concordance rate in monozygotic than in dizygotic twin pairs if one of the twins is diagnosed as schizophrenic. That constitutional weaknesses exist is suggested by data indicating that schizophrenic mothers have a higher incidence of deviant fetal growth in terms of perinatal mortality and malformations in the newborn. Heath has suggested that brain cell antibodies attach themselves to the septal region and impair synaptic transmission there. Areas of investigation now most actively pursued are concerned with the intermediate metabolism of cerebral glucose.

272. **B.** Primary symptoms of schizophrenia include: loosening of associations, autism, ambivalence that dominates the affective life of the patient, and inappropriate affect. Among the secondary symptoms are: delusions and hallucinations. Free association is a technique used in psychoanalytic therapy.

273. **D.** It has been postulated that the parental investment in the child is disturbed from the beginning. That deprivation of early mothering may bring about enduring defects in the capacity to socialize or even to carry out sexual activities effectively now has received strong support from studies in primates and mammalian species. Bateson put forth the hypothesis that the origins of the schizophrenic defects in communication rest upon a "double bind" transaction between two persons. Failure to acquire social skills early narrows the probability of acquisition of emotional relations with extrafamily members in adolescence and adulthood. This limits perceptual discrimination.

274. **A.** Process schizophrenia is attributed more to organic factors than to environmental ones; typically it begins gradually, continues chronically, and progresses (either rapidly or slowly) to an irreversible psychosis.

275. **A.** Sullivan's idea was that some degree of interpersonal relatedness is maintained throughout life by everyone, including the schizophrenic. Whatever had befallen the patient was related to his life experience with a small number of people.

276. **C.** A common early symptom is an aloofness, a withdrawal behind barriers to an area in which would be found loneliness, hopelessness, hatred and fear. The patient does not empathize with the feelings of others and manifests little concern about the realities of his life situation. His plans for his future are often vague and unrealistic.

277. **A.** The capricious, impulsive behavior of the schizophrenic is to be looked upon as a result of an ambivalence of impulse. The concept of ambivalence, or contradictory manifestations of impulse, idea, or affect was greatly stressed by Bleuler.

278. **A.** Autism is the extreme retreat into fantasy. The person is preoccupied with daydreams, fantasies, or psychotic thoughts.

279. **C.** It must be emphasized that social isolation leads to reduced awareness of perceptual stimulation from within and without; it results in reexperiencing and becoming preoccupied with thought processes divorced from ego control, followed by regressive, infantile thinking processes, and hallucinatory satisfactions.

280. **D.** According to Arieti, the schizophrenogenic mother has been found in a minority of cases and has been overgeneralized. His own experience is that about twenty-five percent of mothers of schizophrenics fit this image.

281. **B.** Lidz identified this type of family which is beset by chronic strife and controversy, primarily between the parents.

282. **E.** Wynne observed that some families are vested in fitting together at the expense of individuation and differentiation.

283. **C.** Laing identified the process of mystification whereby a person is forced to deny realistic data to maintain a relationship or percept.

284. **A.** Bateson identified this interaction process in which one individual demands a response to a message containing mutually contradictory signals while the other is unable to respond to the inconsistent or incongruent message.

285. **D.** Bell and Vogel describe the identified patient as the individual sacrificed to play the role of scapegoat.

286. **A.** A symbiotic relationship is usually a three generational concept. The pathologic mother-child symbiosis has some of its origins in unsatisfying marital relationships: that of the mother to her husband and that of the mother's mother to her husband.

287. **D.** The onset of childhood schizophrenia is usually gradual. Marked withdrawal from people, fragmentation of thought processes and speech disturbances are common.

288. **D.** There is evidence that there is an interaction of constitutional and psychological factors.

289. **A.** The primary symptoms have little obvious link to Bleuler's primary symptoms of adult schizophrenia. They include: seclusiveness, bizarre behavior, and regression.

290. **A.** This is characteristic of the child suffering from symbiotic psychosis as described by Margaret Mahler.

291. **A.** When a child does an unacceptable thing, the nurse should criticize the act, not the child. A child should not be threatened with the loss of affection or be disciplined in front of others. Privileges should not be removed for more than a few days.

292. **C.** In order to understand the feelings and reactions to clinical situations that stall the therapeutic process, the nurse must develop the art of identifying and describing her own thoughts and feelings. The nurse then gains perspective and control of the situation.

293. **A.** Paranoia is a chronic mental disorder characterized by persistent, unalterable, systematized, logically reasoned delusions.

294. **D.** Delusions in the schizophrenic often serve rather effectively in subjectively reorganizing his life situations and in dealing with such problems as thwarted drives, frustrated hopes, biological inadequacies, feelings of insecurity, disowned qualities, and gnawing feelings of guilt. The patient's problems, wishes, and conflicts are dramatized and symbolized in fantastic and bizarre forms. There is a tendency for delusions to center around themes of persecution, grandiosity, and/or sex.

295. **A.** Everyone is prone to develop comforting and other psychologically useful fictions to afford support and security to the personality. Employment of wishful thinking by "normal" persons in their struggle for realization of their hopes, and of ra-

tionalization or projection for defensive purposes, serves the same psychological ends as do the delusions of the psychotic and imperceptibly merges into them.

296. **A.** Circumstantiality is a descriptive term given when conversation proceeds indirectly to its goal idea. Automatic knowing refers to the pathological use of "you know." The person really thinks that the listener knows what is about to be said. Scattering refers to the thought disorder in which the patient's thoughts move from one topic to another with no apparent connection between them.

297. **D.** The basic process of withdrawal from interpersonal relationships is present in all schizophrenics.

298. **A.** Hearing voices is the most usual form of hallucination.

299. **B.** A catatonic patient may withhold urine for 24 hours or more and accumulate as much as 2000 cc of urine. He should be supervised to make certain that regular urination occurs, and in some cases, the abdomen should be felt to see if the bladder is distended.

300. **B.** Repression and loneliness are dissociated experiences whereas aloneness and suppression are on the conscious level.

301. **D.** They are defense mechanisms that explain failure, absolve one from blame for the inability to adjust, and attribute one's own hatred to others. Delusions of grandeur would be compensatory.

302. **C.** The drive components are repressed homosexual drives directed toward sexual gratification and power and dependency motivations directed toward gratification of the need for self-esteem and the need to be dependent.

303. **A.** A gratifying interpersonal relationship is the tool to help patients relinquish delusions and hallucinations.

304. **A.** The catatonic type is characterized by phases of stupor or of excitement, in both of which negativism and automatism are prominent features. There may be alterations between little or no movement on the one hand to an explosive outburst of overactivity on the other.

305. **A.** The hebephrenic type of schizophrenia is characterized by disorganized thinking, shallow and inappropriate affect, inappropriate giggling, silly and regressive behavior and mannerisms, and frequent hypochondriacal complaints. Delusions and hallucinations are usually bizarre and not well-organized.

306. **B.** Catatonic excitement is characterized by unorganized and aggressive motor activity. It is not accompanied by emotional expression and is not influenced by external stimuli. The excited catatonic shows impulsive and unpredictable behavior. He may suddenly attack an inoffensive bystander or break a window. Hostility and feelings of resentment are common.

307. **B.** Ideas of persecution are among the most frequent forms of delusions, occurring especially in chronic psychotic disorders.

308. **A.** People who have strong needs for security, acceptance, and protection are most prone to develop psychiatric symptoms when threats to these needs occur. Patients suffering from schizophrenia are known to have reacted unfavorably to situations in which genuine caring and succor were lacking.

309. **D.** The stuporous catatonic client may stand almost immobile, seldom shifting his position during the whole day. The skin of his feet may become turgid and engorged, with swelling of the unsupported parts.

310. **C.** This behavior may serve as a method of meeting situations too difficult to be met by active, resolute measures. It may be thought of as a protective withdrawal from contact with surroundings that seem threatening.

311. **B.** The therapist should simply tell the patient that he does not hear the voices but he will be glad to listen to the patient's experiences.

312. **D.** Nonverbal communication can be a very satisfying experience for a patient who has been isolated from other contacts. The nurse's aim should be to gradually substitute speech for nonverbal methods as the patient is able to tolerate it.

313. **A.** A psychosis is a major mental disorder of organic or emotional origin in which the individual's ability to think, respond emotionally, remember, communicate, interpret reality, and behave appropriately is sufficiently impaired so as to interfere grossly with his capacity to meet the ordinary demands of life.

314. **C.** Delusions are believed to be formed to clarify overwhelming doubts, fears, and anxieties and provide something definite upon which formerly scattered attention can be focused. Her delusion indicates fear of physical harm that may be related to the hospital environment and may result in impulsive behavior.

315. **D.** The basic concept to keep in mind when having to verbally react to symptomatology and communication that the patient displays is that underlying his acute and pressing problems are his feelings of being overwhelmed. The nurse looks for the reality stimuli creating the stress and focuses on the patient's feelings.

316. **C.** The patient needs freedom to express and test her feelings. The nurse indicates by her behavior that she recognizes Mrs. Cook's need and also the needs of others.

317. **A.** The best tact is to explain and give the reality factors, to be clear and honest with the client.

318. **A.** The nurse listens carefully to the patient's account and questions him about any unclear aspects. He helps him to clarify what he seems to be experiencing.

319. **A.** In cases where it is absolutely necessary to control the person's aggression, additional people must be utilized. It is dangerous for the client to feel that he can overcome the nurse. The struggle must be as brief and painless as possible.

320. **A.** The nurse explains all actions and is not friendly or informal. She offers opportunity for questions and maintains emotional distance.

321. **C.** It is generally known and accepted that catatonic patients are in contact with and aware of their environment and its attending situations.

322. **A.** Part of defining reality is responding to the thought disturbance. Trying to talk about what happens and how the patient feels is the therapeutic issue.

323. **D.** Patients should be in a milieu in which they can exert some control and in which simple social relationships are possible. The nurse supports behaviors that move toward reality testing and assists patients to be more aware of social reality. She makes decisions for patients when necessary and helps patients move toward making their own decisions.

324. **B.** By exploring and telling the patient that it would help to look at his thoughts and feelings about the issues, the nurse defines the therapeutic role and does not place herself in a role with which she cannot be comfortable.

325. **B.** The reality factor relates to "you know" and the nurse makes it her focus with the client. She is attempting to help the client to talk about what happened and to discourage automatic knowing.

326. **B.** A delusion is a false, fixed belief that cannot be corrected by logic. Delusions often develop as a defense against intolerable feelings.

327. **A.** Therapy with the delusional patient involves working with the problems the delusion represents, not with the delusion itself. This decoding of the delusion provides understanding of the patient's dynamics and reduces the patient's need for the delusion itself.

328. **B.** The schizophrenic's withdrawal from people and loss of contact with reality is never complete. Each schizophrenic person still has the capacity for relating to people and some contact with reality. Without further data, the safest assumption to make is that Mr. Jensen may be aware of events around him.

329. **D.** One of the major characteristics of schizophrenia is a profound withdrawl from people because past interpersonal relationships have been so painful.

330. **B.** In a therapeutic milieu, the nurse communicates with the patient within the limits that he can manage. The nurse indicates that she understands the patient's fears of reaching out to people and reflects some of his other feeling tones, but her nonverbal friendly acceptance is more important than what she says.

331. **C.** A passive, friendly interaction by staff is often appropriate for patients with severe communication problems. The nurse quietly offers the patient friendly contacts but does not push them if he does not reciprocate.

332. **C.** In many instances the nurse should engage the patient in some kind of activity while talking with him. Frequently it is best to present the patient with a suggestion rather than a choice. Obviously, Mr. Jensen still needs a one-to-one rather than a group approach.

333. **C.** This behavior can be seen as an aspect of a total social field disturbance, the key element of which is the unconfronted disagreement between ward personnel.

334. **B.** The double-bind is a type of interaction, noted frequently in families with schizophrenic members, in which one person demands a response to a message containing mutually contradictory signals while the other is unable either to comment on the incongruity or to escape from the situation.

335. **A.** The nurse should avoid being overly friendly to the patient. A consistent, yet altruistic approach will reduce considerably the patient's anxiety and instill a small measure of trust toward others. Questions should be answered sincerely.

336. **C.** The nurse understood this statement to be an idea of reference. To merely correct the patient would not deal with the patient's reason for making the statement to the nurse. His reason in reality was caused by anxiety. To deal with the idea of reference as if it were real would be to support an unreal statement.

337. **C.** The incorrect interpretation of incidents as having direct reference to the self is an idea of reference.

338. **C.** Thorazine depresses the production of leukocytes. Agranulocytosis is fortunately of low incidence, probably less than 0.3 percent, and it occurs within three to six weeks after the beginning of treatment. Its onset is sudden.

339. **B.** The nurse recognizes that Mr. Clark is projecting. She does not directly confront him and thus perhaps encourage him to deny his anger. She attempts to focus awareness on that fact that people do get angry and behave in certain ways. This allows Mr. Clark to talk about himself or others.

340. **B.** Catatonic patients may be so withdrawn that they do not eat spontaneously and they may withhold urine. The patient needs to be observed. The nurse's fundamental goal is to establish interpersonal contact at the level that the client can tolerate.

341. **A.** Permitting a patient to continue bizarre behavior allows her to become adapted to it, and she becomes increasingly reluctant to give it up. The nurse must clarify for the patient exactly what is expected of her, and she must help her to meet these expectations if she cannot do so unaided.

342. **B.** Depersonalization refers to feelings of unreality or strangeness concerning either the environment or the self or both.

343. **B.** Effective hospital care takes place when the staff affords healthy models for identification and offers opportunities for clear verbal communication, learning of new skills and development of positive ego attitudes through the support of pleasurable and rewarding relationships.

344. **C.** The nurse's basic task with the individual schizophrenic patient is to bridge the psychotic gap that separates him from people and thus help him back to better contact with reality. The nurse offers a reassuring, interpersonal contact.

345. **C.** It is the role of the psychiatric nurse to define reality. When the patient demonstrates inability to reality test, the nurse needs to understand the patient's world and what it means to him. Being able to understand will then help to gain the patient's confidence. The nurse lets the patient know when she understands him and when she does not.

346. **B.** The patient has difficulty with the symbolic aspect of language, manifested by his tendency toward inappropriate concreteness. He interprets the nurse's words in a strangely literal way.

347. **B.** In fully developed catatonic stupor, the patient may abandon all voluntary forms of motor activity. He may lie motionless upon the bed in the fetal position for long periods of time. He may be speechless, completely involuntary of urine and feces, that is, indifferent to these bodily functions.

348. **D.** It is recommended that nurses avoid an "overly friendly" approach. A certain amount of interested detachment may be more comforting and less threatening to the highly suspicious person than oversolicitude.

349. **D.** The client may lodge a capsule in the side of his mouth or under his tongue and later spit it out. This problem can be solved by administering the medication in liquid form and watching the client drink water after taking it.

350. **A.** The well-regulated and structured activity of a therapeutic institution provides arrangements for the reestablishment of the patient's ego, allowing him to make clear-cut discriminations between himself and the environment and to refix his concepts of time and space.

351. **C.** The presence of a well-marked affective element is of hopeful significance. The presence of cyclothymic factors in the personality background renders the prognosis more favorable.

352. **B.** The hebephrenic patient comes to lead a highly autistic life; he becomes bafflingly inaccessible and greatly introverted and withdrawn. The final disintegration of personality and habits is perhaps the greatest of any of the types of schizophrenia.

353. **A.** The more acute the onset, the better the prognosis for a schizophrenic patient.

354. **A.** The better adjusted the patient's prepsychotic personality, the more directly and confidently the patient has been accustomed to meet the problems and difficulties of life, the richer his interests, the more definite an external precipitating situation, and the more rapid the onset, the better the prognosis. The existence of anxiety and of a clear emotional problem makes the prognosis more favorable.

355. **C.** Whitehorn measured schizophrenic patients' heart rates during (1) a rest period, (2) a subsequent period of systematic inquiry into the patients' life histories and problems and (3) a final period in which he discussed with the patients their day-to-day activities on the hospital ward and other ordinary topics. The emotional reactions were much greater in the last stage indicating a response to the contact.

356. **B.** Verbal messages may be ignored. The nurse may need to get his clothes and personal effects ready, take the client by the hand and state simply what needs to be done. The client is assisted as needed with the nurse's supervision.

357. **A.** The interviewer should avoid witty or humorous remarks, particularly if they are directed at the client, as this person has no sense of humor about anything applied to himself. Irony and metaphor are also dangerous.

358. **A.** Approaches include listening for cues and word construction games. These indicate interest in the client and offer stimulation.

359. **B.** It is a period of expectant listening which comprises the first stage of the hallucinatory experience.

360. **A.** The American Public Health Association's Program Area Committee on Mental Health defined the Social Breakdown Syndrome in 1962.

361. **C.** The patterns are (1) withdrawal with loss of interest in the surrounding world, (2) anger and hostility in the form of resentfulness, quarrelsomeness, assaultiveness and (3) mixed tendencies of withdrawal and hostility sometimes exhibited through echolalia, echopraxia and posturing. These are negativistic types of behavior and can be seen as withdrawing aggressively.

362. **D.** It occurs in many different chronic mental disorders, particularly schizophrenia, mental retardation and various organic psychoses.

363. **D.** More commonly, the onset occurs in a single, explosive leap, beginning with violent behavior or the sudden termination of all ordinary social roles. About two-thirds of the episodes start outside the hospital.

364. **D.** In an organic brain syndrome the greatest impairment is for recent recall.

365. **C.** Early recognition by appropriate arteriography of cerebral insufficiency can lead to appropriate surgical endarterectomy or angioplasty.

366. **C.** Depending upon the degree of cerebral insufficiency, the patient reveals symptoms of an increasing degree of disorientation.

367. **B.** The mental disturbances associated with head trauma are either acute or chronic organic brain disorders.

368. **D.** The earliest expression of disturbance in orientation is to time, followed by disturbance of place and then of person.

369. **B.** Alzheimer's disease occurs usually between the ages of 50 and 60 and Pick's disease occurs most frequently between the ages of 45 and 60.

370. **D.** Although these two organic syndromes are extremely difficult to differentiate, those characteristics listed are more common in Pick's disease.

371. **C.** Indifference and underactivity are typical of Pick's disease whereas anxiety and hyperactivity are typical of Alzheimer's disease.

372. **B.** There are some distinct differences in the brain cell changes of Alzheimer's and Pick's disease.

373. **C.** The biggest loss to the elderly is that of a meaningful role. They must be permitted, and sometimes encouraged, to participate in meaningful activities in order to maintain a feeling of usefulness and to preserve their pride.

374. **B.** One form of protection against intolerable anxiety is the use of fabrications, with or without basis in fact, which are accepted by the patient as actual occurrences.

375. **B.** In somewhat more than half of the cases, a sudden attack of confusion is the first obvious mental symptom.

376. **B.** Between fifteen and twenty percent of all first admissions to state hospitals are for psychoses associated with cerebral arteriosclerosis.

377. **D.** Perhaps one of the most significant and also most frequently overlooked factors in the differential diagnosis of the arteriosclerotic brain syndrome is that of the complicating depressive reaction or the depressive reaction of aging.

378. **D.** All of the symptoms listed, including any apparent change in character in a person over 50 (excluding the case of syphilitic meningoencephalitis), should be considered suggestive of cerebral arteriosclerosis.

379. **C.** Low cholesterol diets probably influence the lipid metabolism.

380. **B.** Coffee has a dilatory effect on the cortical vessels and thus reduces the element of delirium. Frequently, the elderly patient will have had some perception of this effect and will increase his consumption of coffee in the attempt to "clear his head."

381. **B.** Confabulation is the process of filling in the memory gaps with detailed, but inaccurate accounts derived from fantasy.

382. **B.** In view of its threat to both life and future cerebral functioning, it is imperative to arrive at early recognition and immediate treatment of the Acute Organic Brain syndrome with the delirious state. Schizophrenic reactions are confused frequently, but usually they may be distinguished by the patient's clear orientation and ability to retain and recall past events, thus demonstrating effective memory.

383. **C.** Human beings, regardless of their age, need a sense of future. It is important for nurses to believe in an ever-present capacity for growth and change if they are to help elderly patients live their lives to the fullest.

384. **D.** Recently hospitalized individuals with arteriosclerotic brain disease may suddenly become confused and disoriented. Calendars and clocks help orient the patient to time.

385. **C.** Elderly patients may sometimes need help to become more responsive to the world about them. Many times reminiscing reduces the depression of the elderly and cuts into feelings of isolation.

386. **D.** Paramount to helping the aged person is conveying to him the need to be needed and permission to be old.

387. **B.** The biggest loss to the elderly is that of a meaningful role. They need to be encouraged to participate as much as possible in planning their own care.

388. **A.** Korsakoff's Psychosis is one of several syndromes that result from a vitamin B deficiency. Chronic alcoholics are particularly prone to this syndrome.

389. **B.** Huntington's Chorea is a degenerative disease of the central nervous system that results from a dominant mutation.

390. **D.** Although in the earlier studies psychotic reactions were noted in thirty to forty percent of the patients, fewer such responses are seen now.

391. **A.** The patient suddenly loses power and tone of all skeletal muscles and often is unable to speak even though he remains conscious.

392. **B.** Sydenham's Chorea is an infectious encephalitis resulting from the factors which produce rheumatic fever or similar diseases.

393. **A.** Approximately eighty-five percent of all clinically recognized cases occur in women. The onset of the illness usually takes place in childhood but it is most commonly recognized during adolescence and early adult life.

394. **A.** Induced hypoglycemic states associated with neuroses have been observed, usually in women and most frequently in nurses who have had experience with the utilization of insulin.

395. **C.** Although senile psychoses result from the interaction of organic and psychological factors, a cheerful, moderately well-adjusted person who maintains contact with others usually escapes the dementia of senility.

396. **C.** Although any of the choices could be true, C is the best choice; by age 60, the majority of persons have suffered a fifty percent loss of the taste buds.

397. **D.** Rarely are the symptoms sufficiently marked to warrant the diagnosis of senile dementia until after 60 years of age.

398. **B.** The transition from usual old age to senile dementia is usually very gradual.

399. **C.** During the latent period in a preparetic patient, the blood test for syphilis may be negative, whereas the cerebrospinal fluid test will always be positive.

400. **A.** The first physical complaint is apt to be that of a headache.

401. **C.** Males account for three cases out of four.

402. **C.** The most common age is about 40 years. Almost ninety percent of cases occur between the ages of 30 and 60 years.

403. **B.** Both atherosclerosis and arteriosclerosis refer to the psychosis owing its impairment of cerebral functioning to the narrowing or obliteration of the lumen.

404. **A.** Given a positive Wasserman and other evidence of neurosyphilis, one of the most valuable tests in determining its type is the colloidal gold test described by Lange in 1912. Degrees of precipitation show as changes from the normal salmon-red color of the solution and range through a slight change to deeper red, to lavender, violet, and red-blue. The colorless solution represents a complete precipitation of the gold.

405. **A.** With the excretion of large amounts of uroporphyrin, the urine attracts attention because of its characteristic red, port-wine color. The diagnosis of porphyria depends upon the finding in the urine of uroporphyrin or porphobilinogen, or both, in excess.

406. **D.** In 1943 penicillin was found to be an active spirocheticidal agent.

407. **C.** It is of interest that when incorrect replies are made with the eyes closed, there is only infrequent improvement with the eyes opened.

408. **D.** Exosomethesia is the term to describe reporting the touch to be outside oneself in space.

CHAPTER IV

Therapeutic Modalities

INTRODUCTION

This chapter will focus on the various forms of psychotherapy and the psychopharmacologic agents in current use with psychiatric patients. While it is the conviction of the authors that psychotherapy is the function of the nurse with graduate education in psychiatric nursing, it is necessary for all nurses to be aware of the purposes and methodology of various models so that they can interact with patients in a manner that is complementary to the therapeutic model and not antagonistic to it. Nurses are called upon to sustain the therapeutic milieu. Thus they need to understand the values and norms that are appropriate and that will provide patients with experiences which foster problem solving and mental health. Since the process of change is implicit in the process of psychotherapy, nurses are frequently expected to be skilled agents of change. This requires a knowledge of the process of change and of systems theory.

Psychopharmacologic agents are dispensed by nurses; thus, it is a nursing responsibility to know the mode of action, usual dosage, and mode of administration as well as the side effects and contraindications for drugs in common use. Other somatic therapies are utilized less frequently and, with the exception of electroshock therapy, will receive less attention in the chapter.

A. Psychotherapeutic Modalities

Directions: For each of the following multiple choice questions, select the ONE most appropriate answer.

1. The main purposes of interviewing in the nurse-patient relationship are for the nurse to

   a. learn about the patient
   b. share knowledge with the patient
   c. encourage healthy behavior
   d. increase self-understanding

   A. a and c
   B. b and c
   C. a, b, and c
   D. a, b, c, and d

   (13:110)

2. Which of the following statements about gestures and human communications are true?

    a. gestures vary from individual to individual
    b. each culture has a limited range of gestures
    c. gestures may influence others and thus lead to a response
    d. gestures are not influenced by culture but are universal

    A. a and c
    B. b and c
    C. a, b, and c
    D. a, c, and d   (20:61)

3. All of the following are important goals in a nurse-patient relationship. Which of these goals is *most* important?

    A. to help the patient meet his emotional needs
    B. to provide warmth, acceptance, and security
    C. to help the patient learn about himself and his predicament
    D. to increase the patient's comfort and minimize his anxiety   (34:58–65)

4. The nurse who experiences negative feelings about a client is demonstrating professional behavior if she

    A. does not share her feelings with the client
    B. does not act upon her feelings
    C. seeks to discover the reason for the client's behavior
    D. seeks to understand the relationship with the client   (2:5–6)

5. Which of the following are reasons for understanding themes in the nurse-patient relationship?

    A. to find out what the process of the relationship is
    B. to make inferences about the relationship

    C. to enable one to compare one situation to another
    D. all of the above   (27:I:137–38)

6. During the working phase of the interview, the nurse is concerned with

    a. defining the goal of the relationship
    b. observing the patient
    c. helping the patient to talk freely
    d. keeping to the issue

    A. a, b, and c
    B. b and c
    C. b, c, and d
    D. a, b, c, and d   (10:91)

7. An inexperienced nurse in her eagerness to develop a good relationship with a client, is often prone to the mistake of behaving in a

    A. social manner
    B. detached manner
    C. overtalkative manner
    D. probing manner   (18:562)

8. The working phase of a therapeutic relationship is partially determined by the

    A. nurse's ability to isolate the problem
    B. nurse's ability to develop a plan of intervention
    C. ability of the client to face the problems with the nurse
    D. insight of the client about his problems   (18:565)

9. Which of the following behaviors may be seen as resistance on the part of the client?

    A. talking about the nurse rather than himself
    B. attempting to convince the nurse he is well and does not need help
    C. arriving late for scheduled appointments
    D. all of the above   (9:99–102)

10. Which of the following processes is a deterrent to constructive movement in the nurse-patient relationship?

A. identical views of each other
B. incompatible views of each other
C. compatible views of each other
D. none of the above   (34:152)

11. Mrs. Petersen has been late for her last three appointments with Miss Jackson, the nurse. Which initial response by Miss Jackson would be most appropriate?

    A. "Mrs. Petersen, I've noticed you've been late for our last three appointments. Let's talk about that."
    B. "Mrs. Petersen, it seems as though you find our appointments upsetting. You've been coming late."
    C. "You must be very busy. You've been late a lot lately."
    D. "Would you like to meet with me later in the day? It seems difficult for you to get here on time."   (9:103)

12. Which reaction is inherent in the termination of the nurse-patient relationship?

    A. separation anxiety
    B. grief reaction
    C. denial
    D. acting out   (18:571)

13. Acceptance of the behavior of a patient by the nurse means

    a. honestly evaluating one's feelings about the patient
    b. approval of his behavior
    c. acknowledging the patient's behavior and his right to behave as he does
    d. avoidance of retaliation

    A. a and b
    B. b and d
    C. a and d
    D. b and c   (34:51-3)

14. Cues that indicate the need for setting limits on a client's behavior include

    a. the client's behavior is disturbing to others
    b. the client is upsetting himself

    c. the nurse's concern about a suicidal patient
    d. the nurse's feelings that the client is asking for them

    A. a and c
    B. b and c
    C. b, c, and d
    D. a, b, c, and d   (10:47)

15. Which of the following are skills that a nurse utilizes in her role of participant-observer?

    a. to understand the meaning of her own actions
    b. to be able to make inferences
    c. to see the elements of an interaction
    d. to be able to clarify

    A. a and b
    B. a, c, and d
    C. b, c, and d
    D. a, b, c, and d   (27:I:146)

16. Which of the following best illustrates the nurse's professional self-concept as a supportive resource person?

    A. knowing what the patient needs and expecting him to accept your help
    B. acting as a partner with a client in order to help him solve his problem
    C. acknowledging that the patient has some creative ideas, but realizing you are the sole judge of the patient's needs
    D. encouraging independent activity by the patient when you think it is appropriate   (29:56)

17. Mr. Ploski tells the nurse, "I didn't want to go to O.T. today." The nurse's most helpful response would be

    A. "Why do you think you felt that way?"
    B. "You should go to O.T. It's part of your treatment."
    C. "You were feeling upset, today?"
    D. "You didn't want to go?"   (26:272-74)

18. A recently hospitalized depressed patient who has a low energy level and low self-esteem, might benefit from

    A. remaining alone in his room
    B. passively observing ward activities
    C. insisting that he join activities
    D. being with other depressed patients
    (2:131-32)

19. In planning recreation for a professional basketball player, one would *not* encourage

    A. golf
    B. chess
    C. reading
    D. basketball (26:325)

20. Going to a family counselor to discuss communication problems of the family is an example of

    A. role induction
    B. coaxing
    C. role modification
    D. coercing (13:58)

21. Mr. Stowe says to the nurse, "My mother complains all the time. She's criticizing me every moment of the day." The most therapeutic response by the nurse is

    A. "Your mother makes you pretty angry."
    B. "How do you feel about what she does?"
    C. "Why do you suppose she does that?"
    D. "She probably means to be helpful."
    (10:81)

22. Through therapy, a passive person gradually begins to be assertive and becomes comfortable in doing so. This is an example of

    A. intellectual insight
    B. emotional insight
    C. reaction formation
    D. sublimation (2:65)

23. Miss Mann, a patient, is talking with Miss Norton, a nurse. Miss Mann tells the nurse,

"I need love but it seems like I'll never have it." The most helpful response would be

    A. "Love is a common, human need and many people feel that way."
    B. "You're feeling rather hopeless now; you'll feel better soon."
    C. "What seems to keep you from getting love?"
    D. "People here seem to offer you love."
    (10:69)

24. When the nurse offers advice to a client, it is usually an indication that the nurse is

    A. concerned about the client's problem
    B. using a technique of presenting alternatives
    C. responding on a social level
    D. responding in a pseudoprofessional manner (10:80)

25. In caring for the suspicious client, the nurse might help him to learn to trust by initially

    A. having him work with other patients in planning an activity
    B. encouraging solitary activities
    C. providing opportunities that give a sense of accomplishment
    D. demonstrating an attitude of active friendliness (26:456)

26. Mr. Lockwood, a nurse, is talking with Mrs. Johnson, a client. During the conversation, Mrs. Johnson does not look at Mr. Lockwood. She begins to swing her leg back and forth. Mr. Lockwood would be most therapeutic if he

    A. tells Mrs. Johnson he'll return when she feels more like talking
    B. asks Mrs. Johnson if she'd like to walk
    C. comments about her leg movements
    D. changes the focus of the conversation
    (18:306)

27. In caring for the regressed patient, a general principle in initiating care is to

    A. assess the strengths as well as the problems

B. assume decision-making for the client
C. utilize simple, repetitive tasks
D. concentrate on the physiological problems (13:305)

28. When the nurse begins to experience fear of a client, the behavior most effective in maintaining the therapeutic relationship is to

A. avoid being alone with the client
B. continue the usual amount of interaction
C. set limits on the client's behavior
D. reflect on the relationship with the client (21:175)

29. Mrs. Holmes is working in occupational therapy with a group of other patients. She begins to appear restless and suddenly gets up from her seat and begins to pace and perspire. She has been diagnosed as having an anxiety neurosis. The best response on the part of the nurse is

A. "What is wrong, Mrs. Holmes?"
B. "Tell me what you are feeling."
C. "You feel anxious, Mrs. Holmes."
D. "You'll feel better if you sit, Mrs. Holmes." (21:173-74)

30. Mr. Keefe, a withdrawn client, has not been able to go to the dining room unless someone takes him. The nurse decides to use behavior modification techniques to change this behavior. She notes that Mr. Keefe stands and faces the dining room when he hears the bell for lunch. She decides to give him a small piece of candy immediately after he does this. This is an example of

A. demonstration-imitation
B. guiding
C. instruction
D. shaping (22:70-3)

31. In working with the withdrawn patient, the nurse might best initiate a relationship by

A. enlisting the patient's help in ward activities
B. telling the patient when she is available

C. engaging the patient in conversations
D. approaching the patient with brief, consistent contacts (26:167)

32. Which of the following is the most important aspect of nursing care of the patient in seclusion?

A. observing the patient at frequent intervals
B. feeding and toileting the patient
C. informing the patient of the reason for seclusion
D. communicating with the patient (26:174)

33. Mr. Kraft comes to visit his wife. He approaches the nurse and says, "My wife thinks she is going crazy or else she wouldn't be here. I'm beginning to wonder myself." Which of the nurse's responses would be most therapeutic?

A. "She's not crazy, Mr. Kraft. She's neurotic."
B. "Perhaps your visit has upset her."
C. "The idea seems to bother you. Tell me more about it."
D. "Does she usually make comments like this?" (2:26)

34. Miss Johnson, a student nurse, is working with Mrs. Gifford, an elderly client. Miss Johnson finds herself behaving with Mrs. Gifford as she does with her grandmother. This is an example of

A. transference
B. counter-transference
C. positive identification
D. empathy (4:25)

35. In coping with the obsessive patient's negativism, the most important consideration for nursing intervention is to

A. avoid directly presenting something different to the patient
B. establish a relationship before actively intervening
C. be direct and incisive in introducing the patient to new situations
D. avoid discussing the negativistic behavior (18:360)

36. Mrs. Klee says to the nurse, "I feel strange today." The nurse replies, "You are feeling strange." This is an example of the technique of

    A. reflection
    B. open-end statement
    C. stating the implied
    D. restating   (26:272)

37. A nurse can best get a patient who is preoccupied with herself or daydreaming to participate in ward activities by

    A. encouraging her to associate with hyperactive patients
    B. encouraging her to read
    C. participating in a quiet game alone with her
    D. placing her in a group and insisting on her participation   (18:307)

38. Mr. Jefferson asks the nurse, "Am I going to be transferred to a state hospital?" The best reply on the part of the nurse if his transfer is planned, is

    A. "You'll have to ask your doctor."
    B. "I'm not sure, Mr. Jefferson."
    C. "It's being planned, Mr. Jefferson."
    D. "We transfer many people there."
                                     (2:111)

39. Which of the following are possible responses to the feeling of powerlessness on the part of psychiatric patients?

    A. incontinence
    B. low self-esteem
    C. compliance
    D. all of the above   (27:I:139–40)

40. The attitude on the part of personnel, which is most helpful to the manic patient is

    A. passive friendliness
    B. active friendliness
    C. kind firmness
    D. indulgence   (21:448–49)

41. Mrs. Miller, a depressed patient, has begun to talk regularly with Miss Clark, a staff nurse. Frequently, Mrs. Miller remarks to Miss Clark that she "should or should not" have done something. Today, she says, "My husband thinks that I shouldn't call my mother anymore." Miss Clark's best initial response would be

    A. "Does your husband always tell you what to do"?
    B. "Your mother would be disappointed if you didn't call."
    C. "What do you think?"
    D. "I think that your husband's opinion concerns you."   (9:127–29)

42. The nurse begins to recognize that she has many angry feelings toward a client. She finds it difficult to spend time with him. She would be demonstrating professional behavior if she

    A. refuses to care for this client
    B. suppresses her feelings and cares for him
    C. talks with her co-workers about her feelings
    D. consciously attempts to be courteous and pleasant   (2:398)

43. Mr. Peters, a new patient, sits and stares and does not respond verbally to staff or other patients. Besides sitting quietly with him, which other intervention might a nurse make?

    A. involve him in a card game with other clients
    B. look at a magazine with him
    C. maintain a conversation about activities on the unit
    D. use touch as this nonverbally shows interest   (2:112)

44. The primary reason for utilizing family therapy as a means of treatment is

    A. the identified patient is not necessarily the sickest member of the family
    B. the family behaves as a homeostatic unit, each member influencing and responding to every other member
    C. the marital relationship is the axis around which all other family relationships are formed

D. the family needs to understand and tolerate the "sick" member's behavior
(5:106)

45. The most essential role of the family therapist is to be a skilled

A. communicator
B. participant observer
C. facilitator
D. arbitrator   (20:617)

46. The most important reason for therapeutic activities to be done in groups is that this method

A. is more economical
B. insures staff supervision
C. allows for comparison and competition
D. provides stimulation   (26:321)

47. Which of the following behaviors is typical in the initial phase of the process of group therapy?

A. hostility
B. free expression of pathology
C. self-appraisal
D. cohesiveness   (27:I:251)

48. Group treatment of adolescents between ages twelve and fifteen is usually characterized by

a. a one sex membership
b. membership of both sexes
c. a discussion focus
d. an activity focus

A. a and b
B. a and c
C. b and c
D. a and d   (6:II:350)

Directions: MATCH the following numbered items (patient's comments) with the most appropriate letter of the group process that is described by the comment.

Questions 49 to 54

49. "I used to think I was the only one who felt like that."   (30:101)

50. "You really get under my skin."   (30:101)
51. "I notice you start smoking more when you're alone."   (30:101)
52. "Please go on, Mary. We're interested in your story."   (30:101)
53. "What do you think about my behavior yesterday?"   (30:101)
54. "I feel like "Someone" when I'm in this group."   (30:101)

A. reality testing
B. group acceptance
C. altruism
D. intellectualization
E. ventilation
F. universalization

Directions: For each of the following multiple choice questions, select the ONE most appropriate answer.

55. In interviewing the acutely psychotic client, the nurse's questions should be

A. directive
B. non-directive
C. formalized
D. probing   (25:42)

56. The basis of psychiatric treatment is

A. the understanding of psychodynamics
B. the ability to effect transference
C. the establishment of meaningful communication
D. the establishment of goals   (1:44)

57. In western culture, communication has been observed to be

A. equally divided between verbal and non-verbal modes
B. predominantly nonverbal
C. unaffected by class differences
D. predominantly verbal   (33:120–21)

58. Redl's life space interview is described as the participant observer

    A. immediately intervening with the disturbing or disturbed social behavior of the child
    B. discussing the life situation of the child
    C. assessing the history of the child
    D. assessing the child's behavior for a 24 hour period (14:9)

Directions: MATCH the following numbered items (themes) with the most appropriate lettered items (theorists).

Questions 59 to 63

59. Ability to love self and others (24:188)
60. Social interest and non-competitiveness (24:188)
61. Accurate interpersonal perception (24:188)

62. Affirmation of one's will (24:188)
63. I-thou relationships (24:188)

    A. Adler
    B. Rank
    C. Buber
    D. Sullivan
    E. Fromm

Directions: For each of the following multiple choice questions, select the ONE most appropriate answer.

64. The type of therapy in which the goal is the restructuring of the personality is

    A. crisis intervention
    B. psychoanalysis
    C. brief psychotherapy
    D. family therapy (1:21)

65. Studies have shown that the patient who might be most likely to "succeed" in psychodynamic-based therapies has all of the following character traits *except*

    A. a strong need to relate to people
    B. a psychological orientation

    C. an intellectual capacity to deal with abstracts
    D. a tendency to blame others, rather than oneself, for his problem (1:44)

66. In brief psychotherapy, the therapist's role is usually

    A. nondirective, exploratory, and that of a passive observer
    B. suppressive, direct, and that of an active participant
    C. nondirective, exploratory, and that of an active participant
    D. suppressive, indirect, and that of a participant observer (1:21-2)

67. Many people choose analytic therapy because

    A. they want to understand the unconscious components of their behavior
    B. it usually lasts for less than 1 year
    C. they wish to eliminate a troublesome symptom without focusing on the unconscious
    D. it is inexpensive compared to other forms of treatment (10:304)

68. Important factors in the technique of psychoanalysis include all of the following *except*

    A. almost exclusive reliance on free association for communications
    B. regularity of time, frequency, and duration of appointments
    C. recumbent position, usually not seeing the analyst
    D. analyst's emotional activity and involvement with the client (1:11-14)

Directions: MATCH the following numbered items with the appropriate lettered items. The items are types of psychotherapy and their definitions.

Questions 69 to 72

69. The techniques are suggestion, advice, faith in authority, praise, and manipulation of the environment (10:304)

70. The therapist reflects the client's feelings via nondirective techniques (10:304)
71. The therapist helps by listening, clarifying conscious problems, and interpreting preconscious conflicts (10:304)
72. Defenses are hammered at and the client is confronted in order to minimize distortion (10:304–05)

    A. Psychoanalytic psychotherapy
    B. Directive and supportive psychotherapy
    C. Client-centered therapy
    D. Reality therapy

Directions: For each of the following multiple choice questions, select the ONE most appropriate answer.

73. All of the following statements about *resistance* to change are true *except*

    A. it increases in proportion to the degree it is perceived as a threat
    B. it decreases in response to direct pressure for change
    C. it decreases when it is perceived as being favored by highly respected others
    D. it increases when those involved have little opportunity to participate in the decision to make the change (19:125–26)

74. The client, with the assistance of the therapist, is said to "work through" a problem when the client is able to demonstrate the

    A. development of insight
    B. identification of problem areas
    C. reconstruction of traumatic events
    D. successful solution of the problem (18:567)

75. The reliving of the neurotic's past in a present relationship with the therapist is called

    A. resistance
    B. countertransference
    C. abreaction
    D. transference neurosis (1:12)

76. "Acting out" refers to behavior that is motivated by feelings that are

    A. aggressive
    B. unconscious
    C. manipulative
    D. self-defeating (25:329)

77. The nurse's understanding and recognition of transference is of value in

    A. psychoanalytically oriented therapy only
    B. guiding one's responses to the client
    C. avoiding assuming the "transferred" qualities
    D. avoiding countertransference (21:426–27)

78. The character traits of the patient who might be most likely to "succeed" in psychodynamic-based therapies are characteristic of the culture of

    A. the lower classes
    B. the middle classes
    C. the upper classes
    D. all of the above (1:44)

79. A form of resistance in which feelings or drives pertaining to treatment or to the therapist are unconsciously displaced to a person or situation outside the therapy is called

    A. transference
    B. countertransference
    C. acting-in
    D. acting-out (25:24)

80. The most widely used method of treatment for psychoneurosis is

    A. psychoanalysis
    B. psychoanalytic psychotherapy
    C. supportive psychotherapy
    D. group therapy (18:338)

Directions: Match the following numbered descriptions with the letter of the most appropriate conceptual model of psychiatric care.

Questions 81 to 95

81. Milieu therapy, therapeutic community concept (10:111)
82. The DSM-II as a currently used classification of abnormal behavior patterns (20:173)
83. Thorazine (chlorpromazine) prescribed for a person who reports hallucinations (10:109)
84. Treatment of symptoms will not resolve the underlying personality conflicts (10:113)
85. The use of tokens to earn special privileges (23:146–47)
86. Patients behave as others expect them to behave (10:111–22)
87. The therapist decides to work with a school-phobic child and his parents jointly (10:111)
88. A person who holds to a fixed system of false beliefs in spite of logical evidence to the contrary is taken to the hospital (10:109)
89. Insight development is a priority (10:113)
90. An alcoholic "bum" is put in jail on a vagrancy charge (10:111)
91. Changing the deviant or abnormal behavior without concern for its unconscious meanings (10:114)
92. The examination of both transference feelings and real feelings in the therapeutic situation (10:113–14)
93. Use of electric shock therapy for treatment of severe depression (10:110)
94. The use of negative reinforcement to modify symptoms (23:56)
95. The use of primary aversive stimuli to treat homosexuality (23:27)

    A. Medical model
    B. Psychological model
    C. Social model
    D. Behavioral model

Directions: For each of the following multiple choice questions, select the ONE most appropriate answer.

Questions 96 to 97

Mrs. Young is recounting a sad experience and is on the verge of tears when she interrupts herself to smoke.

96. Mrs. Young's behavior is an example of

    A. sublimation
    B. acting-in
    C. symbolization
    D. secondary gain (25:24)

97. The most appropriate response to Mrs. Young's behavior on the part of the nurse would be

    A. "How about putting out your cigarette and telling me how you are feeling?"
    B. "Lighting your cigarette seems to help you control your feelings."
    C. "I would prefer that you don't smoke now."
    D. "You seem to want to avoid talking about a painful subject." (25:24)

98. By definition, a crisis is a short term situation lasting from

    A. two to four days
    B. four to six days
    C. two to four weeks
    D. four to six weeks (1:16)

99. Which of the following statements regarding crisis therapy is true?

    A. it has as its goal, personality reorganization
    B. it utilizes exploration of transference phenomena
    C. it allows the client some dependency on the therapist
    D. it is most effective when initiated six weeks following the precipitating event (1:22)

100. The precipitating event or the first stage of a crisis might be

    a. an auto collision
    b. the death of a spouse
    c. discharge from a hospital
    d. the birth of a child

    A. a and b
    B. b only
    C. b and d
    D. all of the above (31:6)

101. All of the following are necessary to precipitate a crisis state in an individual *except*

    A. a severe stress factor
    B. a perceived threat
    C. a rise in tension
    D. a conscious awakening of an unresolved conflict   (1:1)

102. The following are all goals for the first interview in crisis intervention *except*

    A. indentification of the precipitating stress
    B. reduction of the client's anxiety level
    C. formulation of guidelines for action
    D. integration of new coping skills by the client   (31:6)

103. Crisis intervention as a treatment modality has most significantly improved psychiatric care for

    A. the middle sociocultural classes
    B. the lower sociocultural classes
    C. the senior citizen
    D. the adolescent and young adult   (1:48–53)

104. Crisis theory is based on the theory of

    a. Freud
    b. Hartmann
    c. Rado
    d. Erikson
    e. Lindemann
    f. Caplan

    A. a and d
    B. a, c, and d
    C. e and f
    D. all of the above   (1:2)

105. Crisis intervention relies most heavily on which of the following?

    A. the prescriptive approach
    B. the problem-solving approach
    C. the introspective approach
    D. the analytic approach   (1:55–65)

106. An example of a developmental crisis is

    A. loss of a job
    B. diagnosis of multiple sclerosis
    C. divorce from one's spouse
    D. menopausal depression   (1:106)

107. Kubler-Ross has noted which of the following sequences of emotional states as the usual response to one's news of a fatal illness?

    A. shock, anger, denial, depression, bargaining, and acceptance
    B. shock, denial, anger, bargaining, depression, and acceptance
    C. denial, anger, bargaining, acceptance, shock, and depression
    D. acceptance, bargaining, shock, denial, anger, and depression   (32:11)

108. All of the following are reasons why crisis intervention tends to work well as a treatment modality for those in lower sociocultural classes *except*

    A. it can fulfill needs for immediate problem solving
    B. it is direct and short term
    C. the therapist's role is a passive one
    D. no attempt is made to produce drastic behaviorial changes   (1:53)

109. Which of the following is a possible end result of crisis?

    A. the person solves the problem
    B. the person regresses
    C. the person learns to live with the problem
    D. all of the above   (30:44)

110. All of the following are necessary in order for a crisis to be successfully resolved *except*

    A. decrease in anxiety
    B. verbal catharsis
    C. redefinition of the situation
    D. transference   (32:4–9)

111. The key concepts in crisis counseling include all of the following *except*

    A. immediate availability to the client
    B. quick assessment of his emergency situation
    C. purposeful, focused activity that guides him toward adaptive coping
    D. solving the client's problem for him
    (31:33–4)

112. To be effective in intervening in a suicidal crisis, the nurse needs to

    a. assess the lethality of the suicide plan
    b. actively show her concern
    c. point out the client's ambivalence and suggest he does not really want to die
    d. agree with the client's analysis of the situation

    A. a and b
    B. a, b, and c
    C. b, c, and d
    D. a, b, c, and d
    (31:107)

113. Crisis intervention by emergency teams is most likely to fail due to the fact that

    A. triage function is not properly carried out; priorities for handling a massive disaster are inadequately established
    B. team members are so overwhelmed by the psychological aspects that they fail to deal with the physical aspects
    C. staff members are leery of functioning up to the level of their capacity
    D. personal feelings of the staff are blunted or cut off
    (31:15)

114. A person in crisis is an example of openness to change due to

    A. provisional involvement
    B. acceptance of ambivalence
    C. intolerable status quo
    D. removal of critical obstacles
    (19:127)

115. All of the following are appropriate nursing interventions when working with *acutely* suicidal persons *except* planning to

    A. evaluate the client's sense of despair
    B. confront the client with the possible consequences of self-destructive behavior
    C. interpret the meaning of suicidal gestures
    D. observe the client continuously or at very frequent intervals
    (1:22)

116. Which of the following statements regarding milieu therapy are accurate?

    a. different patients need different milieus
    b. the therapeutic community is one type of milieu therapy
    c. in order to understand the effectiveness of milieu therapy, one needs to understand systems theory
    d. the emphasis is on the patient's current weaknesses and liabilities

    A. a and b
    B. a, b, and c
    C. a, c, and d
    D. a, b, c, and d
    (27:II:309–10)

117. Ward X has eighty psychiatric patients. Miss Taylor and Miss Potts want to plan some activities. Which of the following plans are most therapeutic?

    A. select an activity in which all can participate
    B. include only patients who wish to attend
    C. divide the ward into smaller, supervised groups for activities
    D. take a small group of patients off the unit so that others will not feel slighted
    (2:386)

118. Remotivation therapy requires

    a. professional staff
    b. active support of the administration
    c. high information levels for the leader
    d. inservice preparation for the leader

A. a and c
B. a, b, and c
C. b and d
D. a, b, c, and d   (27:II:309–10)

119. Which of the following statements about hypnosis is *not* accurate?

A. above average intelligence and a moderately strong ego are assets to this process
B. usually the subject cannot be induced to violate his habitual standards of conduct
C. it is a technique and not a treatment in itself
D. the hypnotist must terminate the trance state or it will persist indefinitely
          (21:428)

120. Which quality of the nurse is considered of greatest importance in working with emotionally disturbed children?

A. a listening attitude
B. matter of factness
C. emotional warmth
D. emotional distance   (2:459)

121. Theorists with a behavioristic view of man include

a. Thorndike
b. Watson
c. Maslow
d. Skinner

A. a and d
B. a, b, and d
C. c and d
D. d only   (24:191–92)

122. Operant behaviors are usually

a. voluntary activities
b. involuntary activities
c. elicited by preceding events
d. affected by events following them

A. a and c
B. a and d
C. b and c
D. b and d   (2:13–14)

123. Which of the following techniques are most effective in insuring a durable behavioral change?

a. continuous reinforcement schedule
b. variable ratio schedule
c. variable intermittent schedule
d. fading

A. a and d
B. b and c
C. c and d
D. a only   (22:103)

124. Which of the following involve contingent relationships between the occurrence of behavior and the presentation or removal of some consequence?

A. aversive stimulation
B. extinction
C. withdrawal of positive reinforcement
D. reinforcing other behavior   (22:171)

125. The Positive Reinforcement procedure must include

a. events that result in the acceleration of a desired behavior
b. assessing the client's preferences
c. a planned, contingent S-R
d. events that elicit behavior

A. a and b
B. c and d
C. a, b, and c
D. b, c, and d   (22:45)

126. Techniques that accelerate the desired behavior include

a. positive reinforcement
b. negative reinforcement
c. aversion stimulation
d. continuous reinforcement schedule

A. a and d
B. a and b
C. a, b, and c
D. a, b, and d   (22:39–40, 100)

127. Which of the following elements are included in systematic desensitization?

   a. relaxation techniques
   b. assessing the elements of the stimulus
   c. arranging the stimulus behavior into a hierarchy
   d. associating the stimulus with a painful response

   A. a and b
   B. b, c, and d
   C. a and c
   D. a, b, and c   (22:16–17)

128. Generalized-acquired reinforcers include

   a. money
   b. praise
   c. food
   d. attention

   A. a and b
   B. a, b, and c
   C. a, b, and d
   D. a, b, c, and d   (22:53)

129. The nurse would be utilizing the technique of behavior modification therapy known as extinction when she

   A. ignores a response made by a client
   B. chastises a client for his response
   C. rewards a client for his response
   D. models a response for the client (14:112)

130. Aversive conditioning is an appropriate treatment for homosexuality when the factor(s) involved include

   A. anxiety about physical closeness with women
   B. interpersonal anxiety especially with women
   C. positive erotic reactions toward men
   D. all of the above   (6I:951)

131. Maxwell Jones views the nursing role in the therapeutic community as one of

   a. setting limits on behaviors which violate the basic rules of health or safety
   b. interacting with their patients in social situations
   c. helping to transmit the unit culture and philosophy of treatment to the patient
   d. being non-disciplinarian and neutral in their attitude

   A. a and c
   B. b, c, and d
   C. a, b, and c
   D. a, b, and d   (18:385)

132. The concept of a therapeutic community includes which of the following factors?

   a. the current social behavior of the patient is the focus
   b. the patient is an active participant in his own treatment
   c. psychodynamic insights of personality are emphasized
   d. the psychopathology of the patient is the focus

   A. a and b
   B. a and c
   C. b and c
   D. b and d   (10:316)

133. Which was the first therapeutic social clinic in the United States?

   A. Cassell House
   B. Henry Street Settlement
   C. Fountain House
   D. Daytop Lodge   (13:86)

134. Mrs. Jensen, a nurse, makes a home visit to follow up Mr. Ingalls, a discharged client with a diagnosis of schizophrenia, chronic, undifferentiated type. She notes that Mr. Ingalls' mother spends all her time at home and is apprehensive to leave her son alone as he has no friends and nothing to do. One intervention that Mrs. Jensen might appropriately make would be to

A. suggest Mrs. Ingalls go out at least once a week

B. suggest Mrs. Ingalls ask someone else to remain with her son

C. suggest Mr. Ingalls attend the day hospital program

D. support Mrs. Ingalls in her behavior

(21:466)

135. Which of the following statements regarding social class and psychiatric treatment are true?

   a. the higher the socioeconomic status of the client, the greater the probability of discharge from the hospital

   b. the higher the socioeconomic status of the client, the longer the client is likely to be treated on an out-patient basis

   c. the lower the socioeconomic status of the client, the more likely the client will be treated on an out-patient basis

   d. the lower the socioeconomic status of the client, the more likely the client will be isolated from informal groupings in the community

A. a and b
B. b and c
C. a and d
D. a, b, and d

(18:487)

136. Which of the following presents the most difficulty to the psychiatric patient in terms of adaptation and adjustment?

A. hospitalization
B. social isolation
C. discharge
D. job training

(13:178)

137. The nurse might best break the cycle of the "revolving door" phenomenon if

A. visits were made to the home during hospitalization

B. half-way houses were used before final discharge

C. clients were educated about psychiatric medications

D. clients made week-end visits before the final discharge

(13:318–20)

138. Mr. Stevens is employed and lives alone in a single room. He has been seen at the mental health center and is considered to be withdrawn and delusional. The nurse would probably decide that Mr. Stevens would most benefit from

A. full-time hospitalization
B. a day hospital
C. a night hospital
D. out-patient therapy

(21:466)

Directions: Match the number of the description with the letter of the most appropriate organization.

Questions 139 to 145

139. Uses religious approach   (12:148)

140. Residential program staffed largely by former addicts but also uses professionals

(11:272)

141. Provides information and counseling about jobs   (32:336)

142. For spouses of alcoholics   (12:148)

143. First residential facility, managed by former addicts, founded in 1958 in California

(11:270)

144. For teenage children of alcoholics   (12:148)

145. Self-help unit at Lexington, Kentucky

(11:269)

A. Synanon
B. Alanon
C. Matrix House
D. Alcoholics Anonymous
E. Al-teen
F. Odyssey House
G. D.V.R.

Directions: For each of the following multiple choice questions, select the ONE most appropriate answer.

Questions 146 to 151

Mrs. Moore has just learned that her 42-year-old husband has been having an affair with his 26-year-old secretary. She comes into the Community Mental Health Center in a state of anxiety, confusion, and despair.

146. While watching the nurse take an orderly history, Mrs. Moore sees her bring logical order to what seemed a chaotic situation. Mrs. Moore's perception of the nurse's ability to cope, can be described as

    A. ego borrowing
    B. negative identification
    C. pseudoconfidentiality
    D. social regulation   (32:6)

147. According to Beebe, the second step of crisis intervention, understanding the development of the crisis, involves

    A. finding the sequence of events
    B. structuring the interview
    C. avoiding the dangers of premature catharsis
    D. all of the above   (32:6)

148. The experienced nurse therapist can help Mrs. Moore from prematurely expressing her overwhelming emotions about the experience by

    A. identifying with Mrs. Moore
    B. using exclusively nondirective techniques
    C. suggesting hospitalization
    D. maintaining adequate structure and distance in the interview   (32:6–7)

149. Mrs. Moore tells the nurse that she is so upset, she has been thinking of "just ending it all." In assessing Mrs. Moore's suicidal potential, it is most important for the nurse to be

    A. calm and gentle
    B. direct and specific
    C. indirect and general
    D. warm and understanding   (1:59)

150. During the interview, Mrs. Moore begins to cry saying, "How could he do this to me? I've tried to be a good wife." The most appropriate response on the part of the nurse would be

    A. "You must be feeling pretty angry at your husband right now."
    B. "What do you think you might have done to provoke this behavior"?
    C. "Have you ever met your husband's secretary"?
    D. "I can understand what you must be feeling."   (25:186–87)

151. Miss Fallon, a student nurse, is walking down the corridor when John, a tall, heavyset patient comes up behind her, throws his arms around her and kisses her saying, "I like you Miss Fallon." The most appropriate initial response by the student would be to say

    A. "Take your hands off of me."
    B. "Don't do that John; you frightened me."
    C. "Your behavior is very inappropriate for a nurse-patient relationship, John."
    D. "If you ever do that again, I'm going to report it to your doctor."   (21:77)

152. The nurse's approach to the patient who is mentally ill should depend *primarily* on the patient's

    A. age
    B. diagnosis
    C. education
    D. behavior   (21:1)

153. The characteristic of a therapeutic community which seems to make nurses the most uncomfortable is

    A. the amount of time set aside for daily meetings

B. the change in the power structure of the ward

C. the utilization of an open-door policy

D. the increase in the number of patients who go out to work (28:117–18)

154. The assessment technique used by the psychologist which allows the patient the greatest degree of freedom for projection is the

A. interview

B. sentence-completion test

C. Wechsler adult intelligence scale (WAIS)

D. Rorschach test (20:164–66)

155. In deciding whether a depressed patient should be hospitalized or treated with drugs on an outpatient basis, it is *most* important to remember that

A. patients receiving long-term drug therapy, frequently fail to take their medication regularly

B. it is usually necessary for a relative or a "significant other" to help supervise the administration of drugs for this type of patient

C. a normal 10 to 14 day supply of an anti-depressant drug can be fatal if taken at one time

D. it is necessary for a patient to ask his primary physician for a prescription renewal in order to obtain additional medication (31:82)

156. A major difference between behavioral therapy and psychoanalysis (and other "dynamic" therapies) is the emphasis on changing behavior through rewards and punishments rather than

A. assessing the person's problems and strengths

B. exploring the past origin of the behavior

C. using anti-anxiety agents to control symptoms

D. establishing a therapeutic relationship (20:605)

Questions 157 to 158 refer to the assessments of the same client by therapists using different conceptual models.

157. Psychiatric treatment might be expected to *differ* in all of the following *except*

A. validity of interpretations

B. facts considered most significant

C. recommendations and initial plans

D. terminology used in write-ups of findings (10:108–15)

158. Interpretation of a client's behavior using the "medical model" would lead to attempts to change the

A. use of labels and psychiatric diagnosis

B. family disturbances producing a psychotic member

C. attitudes of the hospital staff and admitting psychiatrist

D. neurological dysfunction causing the reported symptom (10:109–10)

159. In a group in which members frequently assume "individual roles," you would anticipate

A. high productivity in achieving group tasks

B. a high degree of group cohesiveness

C. a need for self-diagnosis of the group

D. a high degree of role flexibility among members (28:100)

160. A staff nurse has been conducting an activity group for ten sessions. The clients are beginning to make negative comments about the nurse's leadership. Drawing on the theory of group development, the nurse interprets this change as a possible indication of

A. the stage of group cohesion

B. unexpected group role conflict

C. an expected stage of conflict and rebellion

D. resistance to group change (28:100)

161. Which of the following clients should *not* be asked to join a new activity group?

    A. Mr. Adams, a 68-year-old depressed man with mild organic brain syndrome
    B. Ms. Edwards, a 21-year-old woman, recovering from an overdose of sleeping pills
    C. Mr. Young, a 43-year-old alcoholic
    D. Mrs. Martin, a 30-year-old acute paranoid schizophrenic   (20:388)

162. An open family system might include which of the following?

    a. plan all leisure activities together
    b. function with the wife pursuing a successful career while the husband is providing the child care
    c. cover up the fact that one of the children is a homosexual
    d. accept the fact that the 21-year-old daughter is living with a man

    A. a and b
    B. b and c
    C. c and d
    D. b and d   (20:13)

163. The statement which best describes the behavior of a family exhibiting pseudomutuality is

    A. "Our family fights all the time."
    B. "Mom gets angry a lot, but Dad puts up with it."
    C. "We all feel we have no problems."
    D. "Whenever anything goes wrong, it's Johnny's fault."   (6:I:188)

B. Somatic Therapies

Directions: For each of the following multiple choice questions, select the ONE most appropriate answer.

164. Mrs. Berg is scheduled for a series of electric shock treatments. The most prominent indication for this type of treatment is

    A. assaultive behavior
    B. regression
    C. severe depression
    D. hyperactivity   (20:641)

165. Just before Mrs. Berg is to have her electroshock treatment, (E.S.T.), she becomes extremely anxious, complains of being frightened, and refuses to walk over to the bed. The most appropriate response of the nurse would be to

    A. attempt to get Mrs. Berg to think about something less anxiety-producing
    B. tell Mrs. Berg that you will report this to her doctor
    C. say nothing, but take Mrs. Berg to the bedside
    D. tell Mrs. Berg that you will be there and walk with her over to the bedside   (28:134)

166. Immediately following her E.S.T., Mrs. Berg is most likely to experience a feeling of

    A. dull pain
    B. confusion
    C. agitation
    D. elation   (28:135)

167. Until preventive measures were instituted, the most common complication of electroshock therapy was

    A. fractured tibia
    B. fractured vertebrae
    C. ectopic pregnancy
    D. aphasia   (20:642)

168. Pentothal or Brevital are given during electroshock therapy to

    A. dry pharyngeal and bronchial secretions
    B. reduce the muscular movements of the convulsion
    C. allay anxiety and pain
    D. prevent vertebral fractures   (2:443)

169. Anectine (succinylcholine) is used during electroshock therapy to

A. sedate the client
B. cause temporary amnesia
C. reduce secretions
D. prevent fractures   (2:443)

170. The amount of voltage and time settings in electroshock therapy are determined by

A. norms established through experience
B. the convulsive threshold of the patient
C. the body weight of the client
D. the number of treatments to be given
                                       (20:639)

171. Which of the following medications enhance the effect of the electroshock therapy?

A. Dilantin
B. meprobamate
C. phenergan
D. aspirin   (20:644)

172. The convulsive threshold is higher in

A. males than in females
B. adolescents than in adults
C. black than in whites
D. females than in males   (20:639)

173. After electroshock therapy, when the client is unconscious, he should be placed in a

A. supine position
B. dorsal recumbent position
C. side-lying position
D. Fowler's position   (20:640)

174. Complications of electric shock therapy include all of the following *except*

A. amnesia
B. weight loss
C. headache
D. dislocation of the jaw   (20:641)

175. The amnesia observed with electric shock treatment is

A. retrograde amnesia
B. anterograde amnesia
C. paramnesia
D. functional amnesia   (20:120)

176. During the series of electroshock treatments, the nurse may need to place the electrodes in a slightly different position with each treatment to

A. reduce trauma to the skin
B. enhance the occurrence of seizure
C. maintain electrical contact
D. reduce the probability of headaches
                                       (2:445)

177. Which of the following statements about memory loss from electroshock therapy is accurate?

A. recent memory remains intact
B. permanent memory loss may occur
C. permanent memory loss rarely occurs
D. memory loss of significant life events is typical
                                       (2:445)

178. Electric shock therapy is frequently considered the treatment of choice for

A. obsessive-compulsive neurosis
B. post-partum depression
C. involutional depression
D. reactive depressions   (20:641)

179. Symptoms of delayed reaction to insulin coma therapy include

a. weakness
b. drowsiness
c. profuse perspiration
d. hunger

A. a and c
B. b and c
C. a and d
D. a, b, c, and d   (26:316)

180. Which medication is used to terminate insulin coma?

A. Thorazine
B. Glucagon
C. Indoklon
D. Lactose   (2:447)

181. The major reason(s) insulin coma therapy is not used today is that

    A. it requires extremely close observation during and following the treatment
    B. because of the need for experienced personnel, it is very expensive
    C. treatment results from insulin coma
    D. all of the above   (20:649–51)

182. Indoklon therapy is a similar treatment to

    A. insulin therapy
    B. psychosurgery
    C. electroshock therapy
    D. hydrotherapy   (26:311–12)

183. Insulin shock therapy, Indoklon therapy, and electric shock therapy all have which of the following in common? Each of these therapies

    A. is specific to the treatment of depression
    B. produces a convulsion
    C. is widely used in current psychiatric practice
    D. was developed between 1945 and 1955   (20:639, 644, 651)

184. Which of the following treatments *most* requires highly skilled professionals?

    A. insulin coma therapy
    B. electroshock therapy
    C. hydrotherapy
    D. remotivation therapy   (2:446)

185. All of the following are true about the rauwolfia alkaloids *except*

    A. they came into prominence in the U.S. around 1953
    B. they had been used for many years in India for the treatment of mental disorders
    C. they are especially useful because of their low toxicity in large doses
    D. the most widely used of these compounds is reserpine   (20:630–31)

186. The first major drug breakthrough in treating psychotic patients came about in the early

    A. 1930's
    B. 1940's
    C. 1950's
    D. 1960's   (20:620)

187. Phenothiazines tend to cause which of the following bodily actions?

    a. hypotension
    b. relaxation of smooth muscles
    c. decrease in salivary and gastric secretions
    d. compensatory tachycardia
    e. alteration of pupillary size

    A. a and d
    B. b and e
    C. a, b, d, and e
    D. a, b, c, d, and e   (20:623)

188. Phenothiazines are most often given to patients with

    A. severe agitation and confusion
    B. tendencies toward addiction
    C. extra-pyramidal signs
    D. psychomotor retardation   (10:293–94)

189. The one drug which is historically considered to have had the most far-reaching and significant effects on the treatment of hospitalized mentally ill patients in this country is

    A. Trilafon
    B. Thorazine
    C. Stelazine
    D. Prolixin   (20:620)

190. Mr. Row, a patient at Manhattan State Hospital, will be discharged next week and will continue to be on Thorazine 75 mg TID. When you talk with Mr. Row about the importance of continuing to take his medication regularly, you also discuss a possible side effect which is

    A. increased mucous secretions
    B. increased sensitivity to sunlight

C. decreased appetite
D. decreased acuity in hearing (20:625–26)

Questions 191 to 195

Mrs. Wilkins is a 57-year-old woman who has been admitted to Hawley State Hospital. Her intake interview reveals evidence of paranoid delusions and auditory hallucinations.

191. Mrs. Wilkins is started on Thorazine 50 mg. q.i.d. The nurses caring for her should be aware of possible side effects of any of the phenothiazines including

    a. dry mouth
    b. blurred vision
    c. constipation
    d. weight gain
    e. somnolence

A. a and c
B. b and e
C. a, c, and d
D. a, b, c, d, and e (20:623–27)

192. Several weeks following hospitalization, Mrs. Wilkins becomes increasingly agitated and disturbed. The physician in charge increases her Thorazine to 150 mg q.i.d. The nurse should be alert to such possible physiological effects as

    a. increased sleepiness
    b. decreased pulse and respiration
    c. agranulocytosis
    d. jaundice
    e. drooling and unsteady gait

A. a and b
B. c and d
C. e only
D. a, b, c, d, and e (20:622–27)

193. One afternoon, Mrs. Wilkins becomes extremely agitated and physically abusive to other patients. The nurse administering the stat order of Thorazine 50 mg I.M. should

    a. administer the I.M. dosage very slowly
    b. administer the I.M. dosage very rapidly
    c. massage the site of injection
    d. check Mrs. Wilkins' blood pressure 20 to 40 minutes after the injection
    e. check Mrs. Wilkins' temperature 20 to 40 minutes after the injection

A. a and c
B. b and c
C. a, c, and d
D. b, c, and e (20:623)

194. Several days after this episode, Mrs. Wilkins receives an order for Thorazine concentrate p.o. since the nurses are concerned that she may not be swallowing her pills. When administering Thorazine concentrate, the nurse should

    a. disguise the concentrate in fruit juice
    b. tell Mrs. Wilkins she is receiving her medication in fruit juice
    c. check on Mrs. Wilkins' oral hygiene
    d. wash her hands thoroughly after handling the medication
    e. refuse to give the Thorazine in oral concentrate form

A. a only
B. b and c
C. b, c, and d
D. e only (2:429)

195. The nurse should be *most* concerned about which of the following set of complaints by a patient on Thorazine?

A. dry mouth and constipation
B. malaise and scratchy throat
C. drowsiness and weight gain
D. nasal congestion and unpleasant taste

(20:625–26)

196. The nurse might expect that the paranoid client who receives a phenothiazine for two weeks will become

    A. less delusional
    B. less aggressive
    C. less suspicious
    D. more withdrawn   (21:402–06)

197. A patient who has been receiving a phenothiazine derivative for a month drinks three Martinis while out on a daily pass. Consequently,

    A. in this case, the effect of the alcohol would be more pronounced than that of the alcohol alone
    B. the effect of the alcohol would be lessened because of the phenothiazine
    C. the alcohol and phenothiazine in combination would produce extreme agitation
    D. there would be a marked increase in blood pressure accompanied by dyspnea   (2:431)

198. Before giving chlorpromazine, the nurse should first check the client's

    A. pulse and temperature
    B. blood pressure
    C. pupillary reflexes
    D. apical pulse   (26:363)

199. Mr. Green has a PRN order for I.M. Thorazine for increased agitation. The nurse needs to remember when administering the medication to

    A. check Mr. Green's pulse rate
    B. ask Mr. Green to lie down and to remain in this position for a short period afterward
    C. inject the Thorazine rapidly
    D. have Mr. Green drink at least two glasses of fluid   (20:623)

200. Contraindications to the use of chlorpromazine are

    A. hypertension and hyperglycemia
    B. glaucoma and hypertension
    C. leukemia and cirrhosis
    D. angina and tuberculosis   (2:430)

201. The reason that Artane is frequently given concurrently with Thorazine is to

    A. prevent liver and kidney damage
    B. reduce the possibility of agranulocytosis
    C. potentiate the action of the chlorpromazine
    D. reduce the extra-pyramidal effects of Thorazine   (20:626–27)

202. Which one of these statements best explains why tranquilizing drugs make some psychiatric patients more amenable to psychotherapy? They

    A. produce an increased awareness of self
    B. modify the basic pattern of the psychosis in such a way as to give the patient insight
    C. reduce anxiety so that increasingly deep levels of therapy can be tolerated
    D. eliminate feelings of emotional conflict   (2:427–28)

203. If a hypotensive reaction to tranquilizers occurs, the patient should be in bed with

    A. his head elevated, legs lowered
    B. his head lowered, legs elevated
    C. his head flat, legs elevated
    D. blocks under the head of the bed (2:364)

Directions: MATCH the following numbered items with the most appropriate lettered items. The numbered items represent terms used to describe the behavior illustrated in the lettered items.

Questions 204 to 207

204. Dystonia   (30:96)
205. Akathisia   (30:96)
206. Pseudoparkinsonism   (30:96)
207. Akinesia   (27:II:216)

    A. Constant pacing
    B. Shuffling gait
    C. Torticollis
    D. Weakness, muscle fatigue

Directions: For each of the following multiple choice questions, select the ONE most appropriate answer.

208. The usual starting oral dose of Stelazine for hospitalized psychotic patients is

    A. 200 to 400 mg
    B. 10 to 25 mg
    C. 4 to 10 mg
    D. 100 to 150 mg   (26:368)

209. Side effects of reserpine that limit its therapeutic use include

    A. extra-pyramidal symptoms and dry mouth
    B. depression and hypotension
    C. jaundice and blood dyscrasias
    D. leukopenia and allergic responses
                             (10:293)

210. The nurse should take precautions to avoid contact to the skin with

    A. Tofranil
    B. Thorazine
    C. Phenobarbital
    D. Sparine   (26:366)

211. Which of the following medications are anti-parkinsonian agents?

    a. Cogentin
    b. Kemadrin
    c. Artane
    d. Atarax

    A. a and b
    B. a and c
    C. a, b, and c
    D. a, b, and d   (30:96)

212. The major tranquilizers differ from the minor tranquilizers in that they

    A. reduce hallucinations
    B. reduce extra-pyramidal symptoms
    C. raise the convulsive threshold
    D. none of the above   (2:426–27)

213. Drugs classified as major tranquilizers are also sometimes referred to as

    a. psychotropic drugs
    b. antipsychotic agents
    c. tricyclics
    d. neuroleptics
    e. ataractics

    A. a, b, c, and d
    B. a, b, d, and e
    C. b, c, d, and e
    D. all of the above   (21:408)

214. A person in a crisis precipitated by an overdose of a psychotropic drug might

    a. be found comatose or heavily sedated
    b. appear highly excited, agitated, or delirious
    c. exhibit psychotic behavior and be out of contact with reality
    d. be in shock, pulmonary edema, or respiratory failure

    A. a only
    B. b only
    C. d only
    D. a, b, c, or d   (31:82)

215. Common side effects of Librium (chlordiazepoxide) are
    A. drowsiness and limitation of spontaneity
    B. parkinsonian-like tremors
    C. increased appetite and weight gain
    D. tachycardia and hypertension   (20:637)

216. Which of the following medications has been useful in maintaining the schizophrenic who is inconsistent in taking medication?

    A. Thorazine
    B. Parnate
    C. Haldol
    D. Prolixin   (30:90)

217. Which of the following clients is least likely to respond favorably to antidepressant drugs? One who

 A. feels undeserving of food
 B. awakens early in the morning
 C. believes his stomach is rotting
 D. is unable to concentrate (2:435)

218. A client who is taking imipramine should not take

 A. Librium
 B. Seconal
 C. Stelazine
 D. Nardil (2:437–38)

219. A medication that is used in the treatment of enuresis in children is

 A. Elavil
 B. Tofranil
 C. Mellaril
 D. Placidyl (2:341)

Directions: MATCH the following numbered items with the most appropriate lettered items. The numbered items are symptoms for which the lettered items (drugs) are specific.

Questions 220 to 224

220. Retarded depression (20:633–34)
221. Manic phase of manic-depression (20:632)
222. Depression refractory to tricyclics (20:636)
223. Overactive schizophrenic reaction (20:624)
224. Past tendency to forget medication
 (6:III:659)

 A. Thorazine
 B. Elavil
 C. Prolixin
 D. Nardil
 E. Lithium

Directions: For each of the following multiple choice questions, select the ONE most appropriate answer.

225. If a manic depressive patient who is on Lithium therapy had a serum blood level of 2 mEq, what set of physiological complications would you expect?

 A. none, this is within normal limits for serum blood levels
 B. leukoplakia, agranulocytosis, jaundice
 C. non-toxic goiter, diplopia, oral monilia
 D. seizures, hyperextension of arms and legs, cranial nerve signs (20:633)

226. Persons receiving any of the MAO inhibitors should be cautioned about avoiding specific food substances since they can precipitate

 A. hypotensive crisis
 B. hypertensive crisis
 C. psychotic symptoms
 D. ataxia (31:98)

227. Which of the following are examples of MAO (monoamine oxidase) inhibitors?

 a. Nardil
 b. Elavil
 c. Tofranil
 d. Parnate
 e. Marplan

 A. a, d, and e
 B. b and c
 C. a, c, d, and e
 D. all of the above (31:98)

228. Which of the following drugs is least apt to cause confusion and agitation when given in small amounts to elderly patients?

 A. Doriden
 B. chloral hydrate
 C. Thorazine
 D. Valmid (2:202)

229. A person who takes a sedative hypnotic every night at bedtime could be considered to be all of the following *except*

 A. psychologically dependent
 B. physically addicted

C. neither emotionally dependent nor addicted

D. mentally healthy (2:440)

230. Which of the following central nervous system depressants has the lowest margin of safety?

A. Seconal
B. Doriden
C. Valium
D. Equinil (31:90–1)

231. Withdrawal of which of the following drugs results in Rapid Eye Movement (REM) rebound with frightening nightmares?

a. alcohol
b. pentobarbital (Nembutal)
c. secobarbital (Seconal)
d. imipramine (Tofranil)

A. a and d
B. b and c
C. a, b, and c
D. a only (20:32)

232. Mr. Lee is given an intravenous injection of sodium pentothal. Under the influence of this drug, he relives a traumatic experience of his past and responds as if it were happening again. This reaction is called

A. transference
B. catharsis
C. abreaction
D. dissociation (21:429)

233. A contraindication to the use of disulfiram (Antabuse) is the presence of

A. hypertension
B. diabetes
C. cardiac decompensation
D. liver disease (20:221)

234. Which medication is contraindicated for a patient receiving disulfiram?

A. Elixir of Terpin Hydrate
B. aspirin
C. Milk of Magnesia
D. vitamin A (20:220–21)

235. Which medication is used to relieve the neuritis in Korsakoff's psychosis associated with alcoholism?

A. ferrous sulfate
B. thiamine chloride
C. chlorpromazine
D. paraldehyde (20:214)

236. Methadone (dolophine) is a synthetic narcotic which has which of the following useful properties?

A. it is effective orally
B. it is nonaddicting
C. it only needs to be administered twice a day
D. all of the above (30:160)

237. The primary use of Methadone (dolophine) is that of a

A. substitute for heroin in medical withdrawal of drug addiction
B. tranquilizer in the treatment of delirium tremens
C. short-acting barbiturate to induce sleep
D. muscle relaxant for patients receiving electroshock therapy (20:518)

238. The drug used to reverse respiratory depression that occurs after Methadone overdose is

A. Thorazine
B. Levophed
C. Naloxone
D. Librium (6:III:400)

Directions: MATCH the following numbered items with the most appropriate lettered items in terms of signs or symptoms caused.

Questions 239 to 245

239. LSD   (20:525)
240. Cocaine   (20:522)
241. Marihuana   (20:523)
242. Heroin   (20:514)
243. Seconal   (20:520–21)
244. Airplane glue   (20:525–26)
245. Amphetamines   (20:524)

A. Drowsiness, ataxia, coma, and convulsions
B. Euphoria, depersonalization, and increased desire for sweets
C. Euphoria, exotic fantasies, and a general sense of intoxication
D. CNS depression and hepatitis
E. Sense of exhilaration followed by depression and irritability
F. Loquacity, irritability, and paranoid changes
G. alteration of perceptions, depersonalization, and panic

Directions: For each of the following multiple choice questions, select the ONE most appropriate answer.

246. Which of the following statements about hallucinogens is inaccurate?

A. they have no widespread medicinal use
B. they produce distortions of perceptions, dream images, and hallucinations
C. pharmacologically they are not narcotics
D. they do produce physiological addiction

(13:349)

247. With which of the following medications is it possible that convulsions can occur for several days after the drug is withdrawn?

A. heroin
B. amobarbital
C. cocaine
D. Ritalin

(13:343)

248. The most common cause of drug-related fatalities is from

A. tranquilizers
B. antidepressants
C. narcotics
D. barbiturates

(31:89)

249. Physical addiction can occur with

A. Meprobamate
B. Compazine
C. Thorazine
D. Vesprin

(20:637)

250. Which of the following signs might a nurse expect, on physical examination, from an adult 24 hours or more after the withdrawal from an opiate or narcotic?

a. tachycardia and elevated blood pressure
b. rapid respiration and elevated temperature
c. runny eyes and nose
d. gooseflesh appearance and repeated yawning

A. a only
B. b and d
C. c and d
D. a, b, c, and d

(31:88)

251. Which of the following individuals is probably in a higher risk category from abuse of an opiate or narcotic?

A. a 17-year-old boy with asthma
B. A 30-year-old mother of two children
C. a 26-year-old male with a two year history of addiction
D. a 15-year-old girl with diabetes

(31:86)

252. On her first visit to a new client, the visiting nurse arrives to find Mrs. Smith in a comatose state. Two neighbors greet the nurse and frantically tell her that they think Mrs. Smith took an overdose of medication within the last one to two hours. Select the most appropriate sequence of actions for the nurse to take.

a. arrange for prompt and safe transportation to the hospital
b. establish and maintain an open airway
c. induce vomiting
d. ask the neighbors exactly what they know about Mrs. Smith's medical history
e. try to find out what medication was taken and how much

A. a, d, e, b, c
B. b, c, e, d, a
C. e, b, c, d, a
D. c, b, a, e, d   (31:83–4)

253. The nurse should be aware that the drug abuser often has significant medical problems resulting from or concurrent with his abuse. Common conditions to be examined for include

a. bodily injury, particularly head trauma
b. pneumonia
c. hepatitis
d. localized infections or abscesses at injection site
e. acute septicemia

A. a only
B. c only
C. d only
D. a, b, c. d, and e   (31:88)

254. The most common complaints during the first 8 to 24 hours of individuals undergoing

withdrawal from narcotic dependence include all of the following *except*

A. agitation and sleeplessness
B. fever
C. diarrhea
D. nausea and vomiting   (31:88)

255. Psychosurgery, or the prefrontal lobotomy, was introduced in the mid 1930's by

A. Sakel
B. Meduna
C. Moniz
D. Cerletti and Bini   (20:651)

256. Prefrontal lobotomies were believed to be indicated for

a. extreme obsessive tension states
b. intractable pain
c. conversion hysteria
d. chronic suicidal thoughts

A. a and b
B. c only
C. a, b, and d
D. a, b, c, and d   (20:652)

257. Complications of early lobotomy surgery included

A. convulsive seizures
B. obesity and inertia
C. irritability and profanity
D. all of the above   (20:652)

Chapter IV: Answers and Explanations

1. **D.** The main purposes of interviewing are (1) to gain information, (2) to give information and (3) to motivate. Emphasis is upon relating to the patient and understanding his phenomenal self and that of the nurse rather than cataloging behavior.

2. **C.** Gestural characteristics of human communication vary not only from individual to individual but also from culture to culture. Anthropologists indicate that each culture has a limited range of these communicative acts. Gestures provide information and convey messages to others.

3. **C.** The patient grows in his ability to face reality and to discover practical solutions to problems. He learns as a result of, or because of, the interactive process.

4. **D.** The nurse should examine her relationship with the client to learn something about both the patient and herself. Focusing on herself or the client exclusively negates the partnership.

5. **D.** Themes help the nurse to be aware of what goes on and thus make the situation more amenable to control. They also allow one to make inferences as they afford economical communication. For example, the theme dependence gives the nurse an indication of what a patient needs. Our total impressions are also useful in comparing one situation to another and are more manageable than the full details would be.

6. **C.** During the working phase of the interview, the nurse must be concerned with observing the patient, helping him to talk freely, listening carefully to what he says, and keeping to the issue. At the start of the interview, the goal and nature of the relationship should be defined.

7. **A.** The inexperienced therapist is prone to allow the relationship to become a social one.

8. **C.** The client and therapist have achieved a good working relationship when it is strong enough to enable the client to face unpleasant and painful aspects of his problems and to accede to the inherent demands of therapy to change his behavior.

9. **D.** The client's focusing on superficial content such as current events and staff rather than himself, attempting to convince the nurse that he is well and manifesting inhibitions such as breaking appointments, are ways that the client attempts to protect himself from the potential danger of the interpersonal relationship.

10. **B.** For example, if the nurse sees herself as an authority and the patient as a child and if, at the same time, the patient sees the nurse as a child and himself as an authority, a stalemate to constructive movement exists due to incompatible views. Understanding how each perceives the other is essential to the working phase of the relationship.

11. **A.** Initially, it is useful to call the client's attention to the lateness and explore the possible reasons for resistance.

12. **B.** Grief reactions at the termination of a relationship are essentially similar to those toward the loss of anything of great personal value.

13. **C.** A reasonable degree of objectivity is the goal in nurse-patient interactions.

14. **D.** Limits are needed to insure health or safety needs.

15. **D.** In this role, the nurse takes part in helping the patient to locate, clarify, and solve his problems. The nurse needs to understand her own feelings and actions. She needs to have a sound method for seeking to know and to be able to see the patient's responses in relation to others in a situation, culture, or time period rather than in isolation.

16. **B.** Krikorian divided the nurse's professional self-concepts into three classes: the absolute authoritarian, the accepting authoritarian, and the supportive resource person. Partnership is a prime characteristic of the latter.

17. **D.** This technique has a prompting and encouraging effect and aids in helping the person to focus upon the communication topic.

18. **B.** Sitting alone increases his sense of rejection and isolation. The nurse encourages participation but does not push him. Too many depressed patients have an adverse effect on the individual depressed patient.

19. **D.** Recreation must necessarily be an activity which is different and provides a change from the patient's usual routine.

20. **C.** Role modification includes referral to a third party and exploring to find solutions to conflicts.

21. **B.** Part of the skill in listening to the patient is in using low-keyed words such as "upset" or "uncomfortable" rather than highly-charged negative ones such as "angry" or "furious." When the client feels comfortable with his own feelings, he will choose his own words to illustrate his feelings.

22. **B.** Emotional insight is a self understanding achieved through solving one's problems in therapeutic interpersonal relationships.

23. **C.** This response still supports the patient because he needs to be cared for and it allows him to talk further about his feelings. Well-meaning reassurance, on the other hand, can inhibit the patient.

24. **D.** The nurse who gives advice or makes decisions for a client is taking away the client's opportunity to do something for himself.

25. **C.** Since repeated failures are believed to cause feelings of anxiety and frustration, these patients need to experience success in activities as well as in their interpersonal relationships.

26. **C.** However satisfying the various forms of nonverbal communication are to the patient, the nurse's goal should be to shift the patient from nonverbal to verbal communication.

27. **A.** Knowing what kind of person you are dealing with, his assets and liabilities, will help the nurse to make a more realistic nursing care plan. Looking for the strengths and nurturing these gives impetus for recovery.

28. **D.** This allows the nurse to try different approaches with the client rather than concentrating on the fear. The nurse's own anxiety plays an important role in the nurse-patient interaction and must be examined for its effect on the behavior of the nurse and patient.

29. **C.** The emotions and feelings are generally not available to the patient on a conscious level. One way to offer reassurance is for the nurse to name the predominant emotion that she feels the patient is communicating. This forces the patient to consider, consciously, what he really is feeling by offering a specific concept she may either validate or reject.

30. **D.** Shaping behavior means reinforcing the essential elements of the target behavior. It is essential that Mr. Keefe stand and turn towards the dining room if he is to walk there unassisted.

31. **D.** Brief encounters with withdrawn patients may be helpful in eventually establishing a longer, sustained relationship. They may lead the patient to make overtures toward the nurse which should be recognized as such and acknowledged.

32. **D.** Because seclusion isolates the individual from human contact, it is important to encourage the patient to talk about his behavior, thoughts, and feelings. Seclusion should never be prolonged.

33. **C.** The nurse tries to grasp the feelings of the husband and reflect them to him. This often helps the person to feel that the nurse is interested in him and is trying to understand him and it helps the person to see his feelings more clearly.

34. **B.** Counter-transference refers to the therapist's conscious or unconscious emotional reaction to his patient.

35. **B.** The nurse should develop a good relationship before she makes any demands or active interventions.

36. **A.** Reflection is the return of content verbalized by the individual in whole or in part.

37. **C.** Initially, this type of person needs a satisfying relationship with one person.

38. **C.** The nurse should give an honest, reassuring reply so that the patient does not feel rebuffed or evaded.

39. **D.** Incontinence is one of the defensive responses which a patient will use when he feels powerless. Also inadequate, ineffectual feelings are noted. A person may also comply, thus demonstrating a more rational expression of power.

40. **C.** The nurse's statements are direct, clear, and quietly confident, but never overbearing or challenging. Consistency is of especial importance.

41. **C.** The therapeutic intervention would be for the nurse to encourage the client to describe what her thoughts and feelings are.

42. **C.** When staff members have negative feelings, they must have opportunities to talk out their feelings and resolve them; if not, undesirable feelings of the staff contaminate their relationships with patients.

43. **B.** Activities are useful when a patient is silent much of the time. The general interest shown in the patient is more important than the particular things she says. The activity should be simple.

44. **B.** Family organization is distinguishable from other systems by its high level of intrarelatedness. The family is a unit and thus the actions of any member affect all members.

45. **B.** The family therapist must take the position of a participant observer. At times, she may utilize the other roles but the role of participant observer is the primary one.

46. **D.** The greatest stimulation for an individual comes from relationships with other persons. Common interests and shared experiences are the means by which patients learn to function.

47. **A.** During the initial phase, individuals test limits. They may do this by being hostile towards the hospital, the group experience, or the leader.

48. **D.** Commensurate with one's developmental stage, the opportunity to come to terms with members of one's own sex is a most urgent task. Young adolescents need movement for tension release and they will mediate their difficulties through action more readily than through words.

49. **F.** Finding out that others have the same or similar problems is reassuring to group members.

50. **E.** Group members have an opportunity in a safe setting to "tell it like it is."

51. **D.** Through this mechanism, group members become more aware of others, gain insight, and learn to evaluate symptoms.

52. **C.** This term refers to the phenomenon of group members giving support, advice, encouragement, and love to one another.

53. **A.** Members can check reactions to their behavior, opinions and feelings openly and in a non-threatening atmosphere.

54. **B.** Members have a sense of acceptance, belonging, respect, and comfort in the group.

55. **A.** The principle involved is that the less organized the patient's ego functioning is, the more structure that must be provided by the interviewer.

56. **C.** The basis of psychiatric treatment is the establishment of meaningful communication between the therapist and his patient. If he is unable to accomplish this, the therapist has few alternatives to offer.

57. **B.** Birdwhistell reports that words constitute only thirty-five percent of total human communication. Focusing on the remaining sixty-five percent which is nonverbal has now become an established science.

58. **A.** This interview is held by the participant observer with one or more children whenever it seems appropriate because of behavior patterns that are interfering or may be expected to interfere with whatever activity the child is in at that time. It is essentially a reality-oriented approach.

59. **E.** Fromm stresses the ability to love self and others, the use of reason to understand the world, and the ability to do productive work.

60. **A.** Adler stresses the view that fellowmen are worthy and emphasizes lack of competitiveness in human relations.

61. **D.** Sullivan stresses effective interpersonal relationships and the ability to view others as they are.

62. **B.** Rank stresses the courage to be a unique person, to be creative, and to express differences.

63. **C.** Buber stresses the ability to live in dialogue with fellow men.

64. **B.** In psychoanalysis, the focus of treatment is on the genetic past and the freeing of the unconscious, with the goal of therapy being that of restructuring the personality.

65. **D.** An individual most likely to succeed in psychodynamic-based therapies is introspective in nature and usually has a tendency to blame himself, rather than others, for his problems.

66. **D.** The goals of brief psychotherapy are to remove specific symptoms and to aid in preventing the development of deeper neurotic or psychotic symptoms. Thus the therapist helps the client to focus on the genetic past only as it relates to the present situation, to repress the unconscious and the therapist attempts to intervene psychodynamically.

67. **A.** In psychoanalysis, the analyst connects the patient's inner life and private, unconscious wishes and conflicts with his behavior and his goals.

68. **D.** The analyst needs to be emotionally passive and neutral, specifically abstaining from gratifying the analysand's transference wishes.

69. **B.** Systematic approaches are made to help change the patient's attitude and behavior by encouraging him to accept the values and way of thinking of the therapist.

70. **C.** This entails a structured, permissive relationship in which the "client" aims to gain self-understanding.

71. **A.** The therapist teaches the patient to make correct observations and formulations by increasing his awareness.

72. **D.** The main technique is confrontation. The therapist confronts the patient with the reality of the situation.

73. **B.** Resistance tends to increase in response to direct pressure for change.

74. **D.** Therapeutic work on a given problem is not complete until the solution has been successfully applied a number of times and in a variety of situations. This is the "working through" process.

75. **D.** The principle factor in the transference neurosis is the expression of aggression against the therapist without fear of the reprisal or censure that the patient may have been subjected to by the authority figure in his childhood.

76. **B.** The term "acting out" when strictly used, refers to behavior that is based upon feelings that arise in the transference relationship, and are then displaced onto persons in the patient's everyday life.

77. **B.** The objective of awareness of transference phenomena is the utilization of such knowledge to guide one's responses to the patient, to make them more fully therapeutic.

78. **B.** He is described as a person who needs to relate to people, is psychologically oriented, is introspective and is highly motivated to gain insight. He places a high value on self control and has the ability to accept delayed gratification of his needs.

79. **D.** The patient's behavior is usually ego syntonic and it involves the acting out of emotions instead of experiencing them as part of the therapeutic process.

80. **B.** Ewalt and Farnsworth state that the most widely used method of treatment for psychoneurosis is psychotherapy based on psychoanalytical principles.

81. **C.** The focus of the social model is in the way the individual functions in relation to a specific group.

82. **A.** The Diagnostic and Statistical Manual of Mental Disorders (DSM-II) is the classification of psychiatric disorders officially adopted by the American Psychiatric Association.

83. **A.** The medical model, disease oriented, makes frequent use of pharmacological and somatic therapies.

84. **B.** The psychological model consists of clarifying the meaning of events, feelings, and behavior in order to overcome and master developmental impasses.

85. **D.** Similar to the money economy of the real world, a token economy utilizes tokens as payment for the performance of specified "healthy" or "functional" behaviors by the patients.

86. **C.** Within a given social system, individuals tend to take on specific roles and behaviors.

87. **C.** The therapist may see the client with his spouse or family in an attempt to restructure the social system.

88. **A.** Since the medical model is influenced by the biological and physiological concepts of the body, the psychic problem or illness is frequently treated in a hospital setting with somatic therapies.

89. **B.** The concept that all behavior has meaning and is psychologically understandable is of prime importance.

90. **C.** The individual is expected to be able to function within a family or community group.

91. **D.** The focus of treatment is on modifying maladaptive behavior rather than on psychodynamic formulations.

92. **B.** The therapeutic alliance between the therapist and the patient enables the patient to experience and remember what he has previously avoided experiencing.

93. **A.** The physician maintains his medical distance and treatment is usually of a somatic nature.

94. **D.** Negative reinforcement is an operant technique involving the termination or removal of an aversive stimulus.

95. **D.** A patient is shown pictures of nude persons of the same sex and an aversive stimulus such as heat, cold, loud noise or an electric shock, is simultaneously administered.

96. **B.** Acting-in is a form of resistance. It includes behavior during the interview that is unconsciously motivated to ward off threatening feelings while allowing partial discharge of tension.

97. **B.** The nurse recognizes that although the patient continues the story, she has gained control of her emotions by the interruption and thus her affect is diluted.

98. **D.** Caplan emphasizes that crisis is characteristically self-limiting and lasts from four to six weeks.

99. **C.** The goal of crisis intervention is the resolution of an immediate crisis. Its focus is on the genetic present, with restoration of the individual to his precrisis level of functioning. The therapist's role is direct, suppressive, and active.

100. **D.** Crises may be precipitated by stressful events of special significance to the person or persons affected. These may be accidental, situational, or developmental stresses.

101. **A.** Although the stressor may appear minor to someone else, the person in crisis faces a problem or stressor that he cannot readily solve by using the coping devices that have worked for him before.

102. **D.** The final stage, or crisis resolution, refers to the development of effective adaptive and coping devices. Hopefully, the client will then effectively integrate these coping methods so that he can use them when other problems arise.

103. **B.** Crisis intervention is by no means restricted to those of lower sociocultural levels; however, because of certain inherent factors (it can fulfill needs for immediate problem solving; it is direct and short term; the therapist's role is an active one) it is thought that its techniques are more effective for those at this level than are the techniques of other types of therapy.

104. **D.** The crisis approach to therapeutic intervention has been developed only within the past few decades and is based upon a wide range of theories of human behavior, including those of Freud, Hartman, Rado, Erikson, Lindemann, and Caplan.

105. **B.** A person in crisis faces a problem that he cannot readily solve by using the coping mechanisms that have worked for him before. The person in this situation feels helpless and needs the help of a therapist with a ready and knowledgable competency in problem solving.

106. **D.** There is the potential for maturational crises during the periods of great social, physical, and psychological change experienced by all human beings during the normal growth process and its various developmental phases.

107. **B.** Kubler-Ross has identified the first stage as shock, denial, and isolation. Anger takes place in the second stage with "why me?" feelings. The third stage, that of bargaining, is the patient's way of temporarily dealing with the anger and helplessness. When unable to any longer deny his illness, the terminally ill patient becomes very depressed. If a patient has had sufficient time and help in working through these previously described stages, he will enter the fifth stage, which is acceptance.

108. **C.** In crisis intervention, the therapist's role is an active rather than a passive one. Even those typically wary of strangers tend to respond positively in an emergency situation, to the direct and active intervention by the therapist.

109. **D.** Crisis is not a static condition. The person in crisis will go through stages of attempting to solve the problem. If this is unsuccessful, there is regression. If this is successful, personality changes occur.

110. **D.** A decrease in anxiety, verbalization about the problem, and a redefinition of the problem are all essential for a working through of the crisis. Transference is not necessary since the focus is on the present rather than the reliving of past conflicts and emotions.

111. **D.** The crisis worker helps the patient to problem solve and supports him in this process, but does not solve the client's problem for him.

112. **A.** The first task of any professional in a suicidal crisis is to determine whether the client is physically in immediate danger. The suicidal plan is assessed in terms of lethality, availability, and specificity. It is essential that the worker show concern for and confidence in being able to help the client.

113. **A.** Team members are more often overwhelmed by the physical aspects; thus they fail to deal with the psychological aspects. Staff members frequently attempt to function beyond the limits of their own expertise, thus failing to seek consultation or make appropriate referrals. Rather than personal feelings being blunted or cut off, the worker often tends to allow personal feelings about certain types of problems to interfere with his adequate handling of the case.

114. **C.** A person in crisis is caught in a situation where he feels helpless and unable to take action on his own to solve his problem. Strategies which may be helpful to unfreeze the status quo and begin the change process include (a) provisional involvement in consideration of a situation, (b) direct confrontation, (c) acceptance of ambivalence through catharsis and support, and (d) creating a vacuum in the status quo.

115. **C.** An acutely suicidal individual is a person in crisis. The therapist's role in crisis intervention is direct, suppressive, and active rather than exploratory and interpretive.

116. **B.** Milieu therapy is concerned with physical environment, atmosphere within the psychiatric setting, attitudes, interaction among the staff and patients, interaction among patients, and social organization. It utilizes social systems theory. Milieu therapy is a part of the therapeutic community concept. The strengths of the patient are emphasized.

117. **C.** It is difficult to organize activity programs for wards of more than twenty-five to thirty-five patients. In large hospitals, the activity programs are best arranged for ward groups of this size and a team of nurses and aides is assigned to work with each group.

118. **C.** In order for the technique to be successful in a hospital situation, it must be thoroughly understood by everyone involved with it. It must have the active support of the administration. The leader is trained in an intensive, thirty hour training course.

119. **D.** In the normal or near-normal individual, there is no risk of the hypnotic state persisting indefinitely, once induced. Should the hypnotist leave the subject in the trance state, the latter will eventually fall into a natural sleep and awaken in his normal psychological state.

120. **C.** The ability to be emotionally involved in a warm manner with children and yet to be aware of the ways in which her involvement is therapeutic, is a crucial aspect of psychiatric work with children.

121. **B.** Thorndike and Watson introduced behavioristic views to the United States. B. F. Skinner is the most widely known contributor to behaviorism.

122. **B.** Operant behaviors are usually voluntary ones and are strongly affected by the events that follow them.

123. **B.** To help to make a behavior durable, reinforce it intermittently. Two intermittent schedules include the variable ratio schedule and the variable interval schedule. A continuous schedule accelerates behavior but does not make it durable.

124. **B.** Extinction involves the disruption of the contingency between an activity and its consequences. Positive reinforcers are discontinued.

125. **C.** Positive reinforcement is a method for increasing the frequency of a desirable behavior by presenting a pleasant event, contingent on the occurrence of the behavior. The nurse must arrange the patient's environment so that the desirable behavior produces the positive reinforcers. The nurse must find positive reinforcers by assessment. A positive reinforcer for one person's behavior may not be a positive reinforcer for another's behavior.

126. **D.** Positive and negative reinforcement as well as a continuous reinforcement schedule accelerate or increase the frequency of the desired behavior. Aversive stimulation decelerates, or decreases, the frequency of behavior. The major effect of aversive stimulation is to decelerate behavior.

127. **D.** It is based on the principle that if incompatible responses that inhibit anxiety can be made to occur in the presence of the stimuli that elicit the anxiety, the bond between these stimuli and the anxiety will be weakened. The patient is taught how to relax various parts of his body. The stimulus is broken down into elements and arranged in ascending order from the least to the most anxiety-producing.

128. **C.** Generalized-acquired reinforcers include reinforcers that are affected by more than one source of deprivation. Food, a primary reinforcer, will only remain potent as long as the individual is hungry.

129. **A.** Extinction is the presence of a neutral stimulus. When reinforcement is withheld, the behavior will eventually return to its original unconditioned rate.

130. **C.** Aversive techniques are appropriate only for homosexuals with positive erotic approach conditioning to men as you want to inhibit the unadaptive pleasant excitation related to men. Factors A and B do not involve pleasant excitation.

131. **C.** He views the nurse's role as a tripartite one—authoritarian, social, and therapeutic.

132. **A.** The concept of the therapeutic community, originally developed by Maxwell Jones, includes the belief that the current social behavior of the patient is the focus and that the patient is an active participant in his own treatment and that of his fellow patients. Increased communication between staff and patients is a goal.

133. **C.** It was started after World War II by a group of former mental patients from Rockland State Hospital.

134. **C.** Partial day care is indicated when the patient is too ill to work, but when the home environment is thought not to be contributing in any major way to the illness.

135. **D.** The chance of hospital discharge proved to be greater for higher status individuals both for first discharge and subsequent ones. Upper and middle class patients remained in outpatient care for longer time periods than lower class patients. The lower class individual who has been treated for mental illness appears to remain isolated from formal and informal groups in the community.

136. **C.** Adapting and adjusting to the usual or normal environment after confinement is most difficult. The increased readmission rate to mental hospitals and its relation to the decline in the long-term mental hospital population require close examination.

137. **A.** Visits to the home of the mental patient during his hospitalization afford an opportunity to assess whether the patient is wanted at home and whether the home is conducive to his mental health. There is no substitute for the home visit to assess the family ecology and interaction.

138. **C.** Night hospitalization is to be considered when hospitalization appears indicated and when the work environment is tolerable but the home environment is contributing to the illness.

139. **D.** Alcoholics Anonymous is an organization of alcoholics who acknowledge their powerlessness over alcohol and who turn their will and lives over to a supreme power.

140. **F.** Odyssey House as well as Phoenix Houses and Daytop Village are residential therapeutic communities for drug addicts that are patterned after Synanon. They use such techniques as confrontation therapy, peer pressure, and support development of insight and encouragement of mature behavior. Some of these programs differ from Synanon in time limitation, staff composition, method of support, program emphasis, and detection of drug violation.

141. **G.** The state Department of Vocational Rehabilitation provides help to persons in need of information or counseling in order to obtain suitable jobs.

142. **B.** An adjunct to A.A., Al-Anon works with the spouses of alcoholics.

143. **A.** Synanon has evolved into a communal life style followed by drug abusers seeking rehabilitation as well as non-drug users who seek the challenge of living in an open expressive climate. Once the person is accepted into the program, the length of stay is unlimited.

144. **E.** Al-Ateen is organized to work with children of alcoholics and is an adjunct of A.A.

145. **C.** The Clinical Research Center at Lexington, Kentucky consists of four evaluation and treatment services for drug abusers (Excelsior House, Numen House, YOUnity III, and Ascension House) as well as an autonomous self-help unit called Matrix House.

146. **A.** A great deal of modeling or ego borrowing goes on during this phase of the crisis interview.

147. **D.** Before a person is ready to relive the experience of peak stress or tension, the therapist needs to observe all three considerations.

148. **D.** The emergency therapist strives to give the patient two ways of protecting himself for his overwhelming emotion—structure and distance.

149. **B.** In order to assess the seriousness of a suicidal threat, the questions must be very direct and specific.

150. **A.** The complex emotion of depression commonly includes feelings of anger. The person who feels guilty about his hostile feelings toward another needs help in expressing his anger more directly.

151. **B.** Although the patient's verbal communication is loving, his behavior is aggressive and inappropriate. The nurse needs to set limits on unacceptable behavior. Her open, honest expression of her reason for being frightened would be much more helpful than an intellectual statement of the inappropriateness of the behavior in the nurse-patient relationship.

152. **D.** Although a patient's age, level of education, and diagnosis are all important variables about which the nurse should have knowledge, the behavior observed is the single most important factor in the development by the nurse of a helping relationship.

153. **B.** Careful preparation of both hospital staff and the patients should be assured before a therapeutic community is initiated. The hospital staff may have a great deal of difficulty accepting the activities and responsibilities granted to patients. Involving patients in decision making represents a drastic change in the entire administrative philosophy of many hospitals.

154. **D.** The inkblot pictures on the ten cards of the Rorschach test show a great variety of form and shading and color chosen so that they may have suggestive value for the responder. The person taking the test is asked to state what he sees in the relatively formless blot, what it looks like, what it makes him think of, or what it suggests to him.

155. **C.** In prescribing antidepressant therapy, the physician should be aware that an overdose (consisting of a normal 10 to 14 day supply of the drug) can be fatal.

156. **B.** The primary difference between the conduct of behavior therapy and that of psychoanalysis and the dynamic therapies is the emphasis placed on the control of behavior through "its consequences" rather than its origin in antecedent experiences and pre-existing sets to repetitive psychodynamic response.

157. **A.** Whatever conceptual model is used in the understanding and treatment of mental illness (e.g., the medical model, the social model, the psychological model), interpretations of symptoms and behavior must be based on the facts or data collected by the therapist.

158. **D.** The medical model is influenced by the biological and physiological concepts of the body, the psychic problem having its origin in the functional anatomy of the brain.

159. **C.** In order for the working phase of group therapy to be reached, group members need to be able to share personal feelings and concerns. Group cohesiveness cannot evolve when members are assuming highly individualized roles.

160. **C.** Many groups move from the first developmental phase, or testing period, to a period of conflict and lack of unity, with hostility being directed toward individual members and the leader.

161. **D.** The extremely low self-esteem and the high degree of suspiciousness make the acutely paranoid patient a poor candidate for group work. Because of the patient's sense of basic mistrust and fear of emotional closeness, the patient needs to first learn to feel comfortable relating to individuals before he can function well in a group.

162. **D.** An open system allows for freedom of movement between the system and the outside environment. Thus, in an open family system, it is not necessary for the family to carefully restrict the movement and behavior of the family members.

163. **C.** For a variety of reasons, including the painful experience of separation, there is held to be a strong drive toward maintaining a sense of relation in the pseudomutual family. Even minor conflict and disagreement cannot be tolerated.

164. **C.** The greatest usefulness of electroconvulsive therapy is in depressions.

165. **D.** If a patient is frightened at the thought of receiving treatment, it may be helpful to promise to accompany him and stay with him throughout the experience. Obviously if the promise is made, the nurse must actually carry it out.

166. **B.** After five or six treatments, patients frequently complain of confusion and loss of memory, particularly for recent events.

167. **B.** The most frequent complications in E.S.T. are fractures and dislocations caused by muscular contraction. The fracture occurring most often is a compression fracture of vertebrae in the dorsal area between the second and eighth, usually the third, fourth or fifth vertebra.

168. **C.** Without the barbiturate anesthesia, the patient would feel marked discomfort as the subsequently administered succinylcholine weakens his respiratory musculature and in some instances, the patient might feel the initial passage of electric current.

169. **D.** Anectine is a muscle paralyzing drug and results in weak physical movements during the convulsion. This reduces the chance of fractures of long bones and vertebrae.

170. **B.** While there is a range of usual dosages, the dose must be determined by the convulsive threshold of the individual patient.

171. **A.** Curiously, Dilantin, an anticonvulsant, given simultaneously with shock, enhances the effect of shock.

172. **D.** The convulsive threshold is higher in females than in males.

173. **C.** It is well to roll the patient on his side to prevent inhalation of saliva.

174. **B.** Weight loss is one of the clinical features of depression. Since E.S.T. is used for depression, one would anticipate a gain in weight.

175. **A.** With E.S.T. the amnesia is retrograde. That is, there is loss of memory for events that occurred before the treatment.

176. **A.** Small, circular "electrode burns" occasionally occur on a patient's temples at the sites of the electrode placements; they require shifting the electrode placements slightly on the temples from one treatment to another.

177. **B.** When a patient has ten or more electroshock treatments, he may have a long-lasting or permanent memory defect for the several weeks' period during which he had the treatments.

178. **C.** The most frequent use of E.S.T. is in the treatment of involutional melancholia and in the depressive phase of manic depressive psychoses.

179. **D.** The most outstanding symptoms of a delayed reaction are weakness, drowsiness, unsteady gait, profuse perspiration, and hunger complaints.

180. **B.** The injection of the medication, glucagon hydrochloride, mobilizes glucose from the liver.

181. **D.** The use of insulin coma therapy is rapidly declining because of the cost effectiveness and better treatment modalities available.

182. **C.** Indoklon (flurothyl) inhalation therapy is being used in some hospitals for the treatment of mentally ill patients in whom convulsive therapy is indicated. The technique may be used as a replacement for electroshock therapy.

183. **B.** Electroshock therapy, Indoklon inhalation, and insulin shock treatment each produce a convulsive seizure.

184. **A.** Although all therapies require some professional expertise, insulin coma therapy presents the most life-threatening problems. Evaluating the depths of the comas and the times for terminating them requires considerable experience.

185. **C.** Reserpine is given in small doses with the maximum dose not exceeding 15 mg in 24 hours. Side effects include a tendency to induce or intensify depression and gastrointestinal hemorrhage.

186. **C.** Following the introduction of chlorpromazine in 1952, numerous analogs and other new compounds have been synthesized, tested, and placed in clinical usage. Their widespread prescription has superseded to a large extent, the various forms of shock therapy and the use of psychosurgery.

187. **D.** Fall in blood pressure, slowing of the pulse and respiration, lowering of temperature and BMR, drying of mucous membranes, and general reduction of motor activity are all physiological effects of the phenothiazines.

188. **A.** The phenothiazines are most effectively used in the treatment of schizophrenia, although they may also be beneficial in the treatment of mania, agitated depressions, and behavioral disorders resulting from organic brain disease.

189. **B.** The phenothiazine chlorpromazine (Thorazine) was introduced in 1952 as a potent new pharmacological agent for the treatment of psychoses.

190. **B.** Photosensitivity confined to areas exposed to sunlight may be produced by Thorazine (chlorpromazine). Usually this will result merely in redness and itching, but sometimes it will lead to edema and vesicle formation.

191. **D.** Physiological effects of Thorazine include dry mouth and nasal congestion, blurred vision, sleepiness, constipation, and weight gain.

192. **D.** Physiological changes due to Thorazine range from sleepiness and a decrease in vital signs to the more severe effects such as drooling and unsteady gait, jaundice, and agranulocytosis.

193. **C.** Intramuscular injections of Thorazine should be given deeply in the upper, outer quadrant of the buttock. Massaging the site for 3 to 4 minutes after injection, helps to reduce local irritation. The I.M. should be given slowly and blood pressure checked, since Thorazine causes orthostatic hypotension.

194. **C.** When a syrup preparation is given in a chilled fruit juice to disguise its flavor, the patient should be told he is receiving medication in the beverage and not be deceived. Oral hygiene is important, both because the medication is being given by mouth and because Thorazine causes drying of the mucous membranes. The nurse needs to wash her hands to avoid contact dermatitis.

195. **B.** Malaise and scratchy throat are indications of possible depression of the production of leukocytes.

196. **B.** Outward-directed aggression is usually reduced. The patient's actual thought processes appear to be but little affected by the drug. Delusions are apt to persist. In general, the patient tends to become calmer, quieter, more relaxed, and often less withdrawn.

197. **A.** Patients taking phenothiazines should not drink alcohol since the combined effects of alcohol and phenothiazines may cause drowsiness, physical incoordination, and giddiness.

198. **B.** To prevent the development of serious side effects, most hospitals check the blood pressure of patients taking tranquilizers.

199. **B.** Since Thorazine has a hypotensive effect, it is particularly important to ask the patient to lie down when giving the drug intramuscularly because of the rapidity of the effect.

200. **C.** Jaundice or blood count abnormalities require the immediate termination of the medication.

201. **D.** Parkinsonism appears in about 10% of the patients receiving full doses of chlorpromazine (Thorazine). The extrapyramidal symptoms of muscular rigidity, slowness of movement, festinating gait, pill rolling tremor, are always reversible and may be relieved by drugs like Cogentin or Artane.

202. **C.** The major tranquilizers are believed to exert their main action on lower brain centers. They reduce agitation, hostility, panic, and overactivity and, in time, they lead in many cases to loss of hallucinations, delusions, and abnormal physical behavior.

203. **B.** If a hypotensive reaction occurs, the patient should be placed in a recumbent position in bed with the head lowered and the legs elevated.

204. **C.** Dystonia is manifested by muscle spasms of the head, neck, lips, and tongue.

205. **A.** Akathisia is motor restlessness.

206. **B.** Shuffling gait is a characteristic symptom of Parkinson's disease, thus the term pseudo-parkinsonism.

207. **D.** Akinesia is manifested by weakness and muscle fatigue. In advanced forms, patients complain of aches and pains in the musculature of the affected limbs.

208. **C.** The usual starting oral adult dose for hospitalized mentally ill patients is 2.0 mg to 5.0 mg given twice a day as prescribed.

209. **B.** Reserpine is a natural complex chemical found in the juices of an Indian shrub called snakeroot. Reserpine (Serpasil) can cause side effects that include depression, hypotension, and upper gastrointestinal distress.

210. **B.** Nursing personnel who are in frequent contact with Thorazine may develop contact dermatitis. This is true in handling ampules, multiple dose vials, syringes and especially oral concentrates.

211. **C.** Atarax is a mild tranquilizer.

212. **A.** The major tranquilizers are also called the antipsychotic medications. Minor tranquilizers are called the antianxiety medications.

213. **B.** Tricyclics are the iminodibenzyl derivatives (antidepressant drugs) such as amitriptyline (Elavil) and imipramine (Tofranil).

214. **D.** A crisis associated with psychotropic drugs may take one of several forms. A patient might be discovered in a comatose state or else be highly excited, agitated, or delirious. Likewise, a patient could exhibit psychotic behavior or serious physical signs such as hypotension, shock, pulmonary edema, or respiratory failure.

215. **A.** Librium is a muscle relaxant and anticonvulsant with properties similar to the phenothiazines.

216. **D.** Prolixin enanthate (fluphenazine enanthate) is of exceptional value in the community mental health setting. Given I.M. every ten days to two weeks in a dose of 0.25 to 2cc (25mg/cc), this drug can effectively handle most psychotic symptomatology. It is widely used in outpatient services where there is some question as to the patient's reliability regarding the taking of oral medication.

217. **C.** When a depressed patient has delusions and hallucinations, the probability that an antidepressant will help him is much reduced.

218. **D.** If both a tricyclic compound and a monoamine oxidase inhibitor are given at the same time, or within a two week interval of each other, they may cause serious or even fatal reactions.

219. **B.** Imipramine (Tofranil) has been prescribed in 25 mg or 50 mg doses at bedtime, since as one of its common side effects, this antidepressant drug tends to inhibit bladder evacuation.

220. **B.** Elavil is effective with retarded depression.

221. **E.** Lithium is effective with manic or hypomanic behavior.

222. **D.** Nardil is effective in the treatment of depression.

223. **A.** Thorazine is effective in controlling psychomotor overactivity.

224. **C.** Prolixin can be injected every two weeks and remains effective for a 15 day period.

225. **D.** Toxic symptoms may occur when serum lithium levels are above 1.5 mEq per liter. Initial toxicity is indicated by nausea, abdominal cramps, vomiting, diarrhea, thirst and polyuria. If the drug is continued, central nervous system symptoms of marked lethargy, coarse tremors and muscular twitchings, ataxia, slurred speech and convulsions ensue.

226. **B.** The interaction of the MAO inhibitors with specific food substances cause sudden, severe hypertensive crises.

227. **A.** Monoamine oxidase inhibitors include Nardil, Parnate, Marplan, and Niamid. Elavil and Tofranil are tricyclics. Both MAO inhibitors and tricyclics are antidepressant drugs.

228. **C.** The phenothiazines are the drugs of choice for calming agitated elderly patients as they have less effect on the cerebral cortex than other types of medications.

229. **B.** A person taking a sedative hypnotic only at bedtime, may become emotionally dependent on the drug but he cannot become physically addicted to it. This is due to the fact that his blood is free of the drug, or has a negligible level of it, for a large part of each 24 hours.

230. **B.** Glutethimide (Doriden) is of special concern because it is more toxic than barbituates. The fatal dose (about 10 grams) is only 10 or 20 times the usual nightly dose.

231. **C.** Particularly after the withdrawal of barbiturates and alcohol given over prolonged periods, the increased REM periods are punctuated by frightening nightmares.

232. **C.** Abreaction is vivid recall with the expression of emotion appropriate to the original situation.

233. **C.** Experience with a large series of patients suggests that the only important contraindication is cardiac decompensation.

234. **A.** Elixir of Terpin Hydrate contains alcohol.

235. **B.** To correct the deficiency of vitamin B_1, thiamine chloride is given.

236. **A.** Methadone acts two to three times longer than heroin and other opiate narcotics and so is given once a day. Many people feel that only the addicting substance is changed since an addict needs to remain on a maintenance dose indefinitely.

237. **A.** The addict is considered to need this drug in order to obtain a comfortable physiological state which will allow social functioning.

238. **C.** Naloxone is an antidote to be given repeatedly over a twenty-four hour period.

239. **G.** LSD produces vivid alteration of consciousness, kaleidoscopic visual hallucinations, distortions of body percept, and frequently, feelings of panic or terror.

240. **E.** Cocaine initially produces a marked stimulation and sense of self confidence followed by weakness, restlessness, and irritability.

241. **B.** Along with increased sensitivity and change in time perception, marihuana users report increased thirst, giggling, and sexual arousal.

242. **D.** Heroin and other opiates cause such CNS symptoms as lethargy and lack of ambition. "Mainlining" of heroin results in drug related infections such as septicemia.

243. **A.** Barbiturate intoxication results in emotional outbursts, progressive drowsiness, and finally coma. An abrupt withdrawal can result in grand mal convulsions.

244. **C.** "Sniffing" by children and adolescents of gasoline fumes and other volatile substances containing hydrocarbons produce these symptoms of euphoria.

245. **F.** Following increased energy, restlessness and rapidity of speech, amphetamines can produce psychotic symptoms, particularly of the paranoid type.

246. **D.** LSD and cannabis sativa may create tolerance and psychological dependence may develop, but it is seldom intense; physiological dependence does not occur.

247. **B.** Convulsions can occur within 16 hours or as late as the eighth day in the barbiturate withdrawal syndrome.

248. **D.** The most frequently used drugs in suicide attempts and the most common cause of drug fatalities are barbiturates.

249. **A.** Continued ingestion of large doses of meprobamate can create physical dependence, manifested on abrupt withdrawal of the drug by hyper-irritability of the central nervous system, and convulsions.

250. **D.** The most common complaints of withdrawal from an opiate or narcotic are agitation, sleeplessness, chills, muscular discomfort, diarrhea, nausea, and vomiting. Physical examination may reveal tachycardia, elevated blood pressure, rapid respiration, and temperature elevation. Runny eyes and nose, a goose-flesh appearance, and repeated yawning are also frequently observed.

251. **A.** When opiates and narcotics are sold "on the street," they are frequently altered with other substances so that the actual dose and specific drug is unpredictable. What makes a lethal dose varies according to the patient's age, physical condition, and tolerance to the drug. For example, the risk is greatly increased in the asthmatic patient.

252. **B.** The steps to follow in a drug overdosage crisis are: 1) establish an airway and prevent aspiration

of vomitus, 2) induce vomiting, 3) attempt to identify what and how much medication was taken, 4) ask who knows the person, his friends and relatives, 5) arrange for prompt and safe transportation to the hospital, and 6) if the patient approaches a delirious state, be firm, but friendly in dealing with him.

253. **D.** The drug abuser often has significant problems resulting from or concurrent with his disease. These include: trauma and bodily injury; localized infections; abscesses or hematoma, pneumonia; severe allergic reactions, acute septicemia, hepatitis, and passive infant addiction in pregnant states.

254. **B.** Although an elevated temperature may be measured several days after withdrawal, the most common initial complaints are agitation, sleeplessness, chills, muscular discomfort, diarrhea, nausea, and vomiting.

255. **C.** The operation of lobotomy, a surgical procedure consisting of a severing of the connection between the thalamus and frontal lobe, was developed by a Portuguese neurologist, Egas Moniz, and first performed by the neurosurgeon, Almeida Lima, in 1935.

256. **C.** The best results are secured in patients who show tension, agitation and distress, depression, worry, intractable pain syndrome, compulsion, hostility and excited, impulsive behavior. Such symptoms as phobias, obsessions, hallucinations, and delusional states are relieved if they have not existed for extended periods.

257. **D.** After an initial stuporous phase, patients may become noisy and overactive. Often they must be toileted, bathed, dressed and fed. An excessive appetite is common. The chief complication of lobotomy is the development of convulsive seizures.

CHAPTER V

Miscellaneous

INTRODUCTION

Professional responsibilities, terminology and psychology through literature provide the focus of this last chapter. With the increased sophistication of the consumer and the easier access to mental health services, there has come a heightened sense of responsibility concerning the ethical and legal issues of psychiatric care. Therefore, the present laws and their implications for nursing will be emphasized. Nursing, as a profession, has distinct responsibilities apart from those which are legally mandated. Situational questions have been constructed to attempt to elucidate these responsibilities.

Terminology has been presented throughout the previous chapters; however, some terms seemed more appropriately placed in a separate category. As authors of creative literature have often demonstrated great sensitivity in presenting and describing psychological facets of human behavior, we have included questions which depict these psychological insights.

A. Professional Responsibilities

Directions: For each of the following multiple choice questions, select the ONE most appropriate answer.

Questions 1 to 3

A meeting is held between staff and student nurses to discuss quality of patient care. The students perceived staff responses to their "objective" observations as rigid and defensive and believe that none of their suggested changes will be implemented.

1. A discussion of the meeting in terms of change theory led the students to conclude that their approach was unsuccessful because

A. high-prestige others favored change
B. those involved participated in the decision to make change
C. direct pressure for change increased resistance
D. confrontation is an effective change tactic (19:125–26)

2. As a second plan, the students decide to attempt to form relationships with individual staff members. For this approach, the students need to keep in mind

A. it is not necessary to include every staff member in this plan
B. attempting to encourage individuals to deviate from the group norms will increase resistance

164

C. resistance will be increased if high prestige staff members perceive a need for change

D. change agents should be perceived as outsiders rather than group members
(19:125)

3. After more discussion among themselves, the student nurses focus on one particular situation they wish to alter and offer to work with staff in implementing this change. Which of the following statements is the most important in their subsequent success?

A. the more attractive the group is to its members, the greater the influence of the group on its members

B. resistance to change is decreased when those involved can experience the new situation under conditions of minimal threat

C. the greater the prestige of any group member in the eyes of other members, the greater influence he can exert

D. resistance to change decreases in response to direct pressure for change
(19:126)

4. Which of the following statements *best* guides the behavior of a professional nurse in an emergency situation?

A. according to common law, there is no legal duty for a layman or medical professional to aid a person in trouble

B. in current practice today, there is no positive legal responsibility to rescue or treat

C. the same legal duty that firemen or policemen have to help a victim within their jurisdiction applies to the relationship between a parent and child

D. once aid is offered, it must be given properly
(31:16)

5. A nurse is liable for malpractice if

a. she gives a medication intramuscularly without objecting that the usual method is intravenous

b. a patient under her care needing bedrails does not have them provided

c. she relies solely on a monitoring machine to the exclusion of her own observation and care

d. she follows a doctor's written order when she should have used independent judgement to the contrary

A. a and c
B. b and d
C. all of the above
D. none of the above
(31:16–17)

6. Although written consent for emergency treatment is desirable, the nurse is not held liable for obtaining consent if

A. an adult is incompetent
B. a patient is unconscious
C. a person is in crisis
D. all of the above
(31:18)

7. All of the following statements about the Good Samaritan law are true *except* that it

A. provides that a professional rendering good faith emergency care at the scene of an accident, barring gross negligence, will be protected from future liability

B. is a statute adopted by almost all states

C. excludes coverage for physicians' assistants

D. applies to situations in which nurses are called to an emergency in an official capacity
(31:17)

8. Which of the following are viable alternatives for the nurse working with an emotionally disturbed patient who is unwilling to remain under care?

A. if sufficiently disturbed, he may be committed involuntarily

B. if he is in life-threatening danger, the patient's consent for treatment may be waived

C. if he refuses her care he may sign himself out "against medical advice" and she must record this

D. all of the above
(31:16)

9. All of the following statements are true *except*

   A. a hospital always has the right to turn away patients at the emergency room door
   B. a hospital may transfer or refer a patient when he has been stabilized before transfer
   C. a patient released prematurely can later sue a hospital staff and facility
   D. a patient may be permitted to sign himself out of care "against medical advice" (31:16)

Questions 10 to 13

Jane Smith, R.N. is driving home from work when she comes upon a car which has skidded across the highway and smashed into an oncoming car. On investigation she sees three persons in the wreckage who appear to be dead and the driver, a young woman whose head is bleeding profusely.

10. Jane's decision to stop and offer emergency treatment was based on the correct assumption that

    A. because she is a registered nurse, she is free from future liability for her care rendered
    B. approximately one-half the states have a Good Samaritan law under which she is afforded protection against future liability suits
    C. although only physicians are covered by the Good Samaritan law, she has a moral responsibility to stop and offer her assistance
    D. there have actually been few instances where health professionals have been sued for offering unsolicited emergency aid (31:17)

11. Which of the following is the most appropriate initial statement for the nurse to make to the bleeding young woman

    A. "I am Jane Smith, a nurse. What is your name?"
    B. "Please do not worry, I will find someone to help you."

C. "Try to relax, you are a very lucky young woman to be alive."
D. "As calmly as you can try to tell me just what happened." (31:8)

12. If Mrs. Ryan, the accident victim, asks Jane about the condition of her companions in the car, Jane's best response would be

    A. "I have no idea. I haven't had a chance to look"
    B. "I am sorry but I'm afraid the other three are dead"
    C. "Try not to think about anything right now until the ambulance arrives"
    D. "They seem to be badly injured" (31:9)

13. Jane needs to remember which of the following concepts which are important for the emergency worker?

    A. remain calm and modulate your voice
    B. a slow steady stream of talk assures the client of your presence
    C. the worker's use of touch is both normal and appropriate
    D. all of the above (31:8–9)

14. Mental patients (except for those who have been committed to a hospital by the court) have certain legal rights. These rights include all of the following *except* the right to

    A. vote
    B. drive a car
    C. make a will
    D. sign a business contract (2:513)

15. Consent for special psychiatric treatment of a voluntary patient in an in-patient setting is required

    a. in written form
    b. of the patient and his nearest relative
    c. to be informed consent
    d. before the treatment is given

    A. a, b, and c
    B. b, c, and d
    C. a and d
    D. a, b, c, and d (2:514–15)

16. Which of the following laws defines criminal insanity?

    a. Currens Formula
    b. the McNaghten Rule
    c. the Harrison Act
    d. the Durham Decision

    A. a and b
    B. c and d
    C. b and d
    D. a, b, and d   (4:25–6,32,58)

17. A person can make a valid will if he demonstrates that he

    a. understands the intent of the will
    b. can identify his heirs
    c. can identify his estate
    d. has no psychiatric illnesses

    A. a and b
    B. a, b, and c
    C. a, b, and d
    D. a, c, and d   (2:516)

18. A voluntarily admitted patient who elopes from the hospital can be

    A. brought back without his consent
    B. automatically committed
    C. brought back only if he consents
    D. detained by the police   (2:516)

19. The patient may leave the hospital whenever he wishes if his status is that of

    a. voluntary commitment
    b. voluntary admission
    c. involuntary commitment
    d. one physician certification

    A. a and b
    B. b only
    C. a, b, and d
    D. a, b, c, and d   (4:20)

20. The legally committed patient has the right to

    a. conduct business
    b. vote
    c. terminate treatment
    d. consult an attorney

    A. b and d
    B. a and c
    C. a, b, and d
    D. b and d   (2:513)

21. Which of the following states have laws making nurse-patient relationships privileged?

    a. Arkansas
    b. California
    c. New Jersey
    d. Pennsylvania

    A. a
    B. b and c
    C. a and b
    D. a, b, c, and d   (2:523)

B. Terminology

Directions: MATCH the following numbered items with the most appropriate role (lettered items).

Questions 22 to 31

22. Susie is the "mother" in playing house   (13:57–8)
23. John passes state boards as a registered nurse   (13:57)
24. Mary decides to befriend Paula   (13:57)
25. Mr. Jones is a senior citizen   (13:57)
26. Peter is "Lincoln" in the high school play   (13:57–8)
27. Pattie has her fifth birthday   (13:57)
28. Louise is elected class president   (13:57)
29. Mrs. Patterson has her first baby   (13:57)
30. Two student nurses role play   (13:57–8)
31. Thomas protects his brother from bullies   (13:57)

    A. Ascribed role
    B. Achieved role
    C. Adopted role
    D. Assumed role

Directions: For each of the following multiple choice questions, select the ONE most appropriate answer.

32. Psychiatry is concerned with feelings, thinking, and interpersonal relationships that are

    A. normal
    B. disordered
    C. normal or disordered
    D. unconscious   (2:65)

33. Cathexis refers to

    A. the opportunity to express thoughts, feelings, and perceptions
    B. the emotional investment in a person, object, or idea
    C. that which takes place within the mind
    D. an undertaking that involves activity, energy, and courage   (10:410)

34. When the nurse *unconsciously* masks sad feelings with cheerful ones while in the presence of a dying patient, the nurse's communication can be said to be

    A. metacommunication
    B. pseudocommunication
    C. a double-bind type
    D. mystifying   (33:122–23)

35. Which of the following statements concerning functional psychiatric disorders is true?

    A. functional disorders are characterized by abrupt onsets
    B. functional disorders are clearly observable by mid-adolescence
    C. the earlier the original psychological trauma, the more severe the disorder type will be
    D. The earlier the symptoms occur, the less likely the recovery, regardless of intervention   (21:271)

36. Mr. Thomas turns to the opposite side of his bed to give Mr. Jason, the patient in the next bed, some sense of privacy while Mrs. Jason visits. This is an example of

    A. selective inattention
    B. territoriality
    C. civil inattention
    D. projective identification   (33:263)

37. Ataraxy is the opposite of

    A. cataplexy
    B. catalepsy
    C. anxiety
    D. agnosia   (4:13)

38. Knowing that one's dislike of a new acquaintance is related to an unpleasant occurrence in one's past is most accurately termed

    A. cognition
    B. perception
    C. apperception
    D. prejudice   (7:119)

39. The patient who unconsciously takes on characteristics of a favorite movie idol is demonstrating

    A. hero worship
    B. appersonification
    C. positive transference
    D. delusions of grandeur   (7:119)

40. The analytic rule refers to the

    A. use of free association
    B. resolution of unconscious conflict
    C. use of the non-directive approach
    D. use of the couch   (7:82)

41. A synonym for obsessive compulsive personality is

    A. borderline personality
    B. anankastic personality
    C. perfectionistic personality
    D. explosive personality   (7:82)

Directions: MATCH the number of the descriptive phenomena with the letter of the correct term.

Questions 42 to 45

42. Our interpretations of what others think of us (5:40)
43. The tendency of a system to maintain structure (5:19)
44. The relief of systems due to the belief that the prescribed substance has indeed been a medication (4:74)
45. Increased motivation and productivity due to being the subject in a study (5:60)

    A. Placebo effect
    B. "Looking glass self" effect
    C. Hawthorne effect
    D. Morphostatic effect

Directions: For each of the following multiple choice questions, selct the ONE most appropriate answer.

46. Adjustment refers to the

    A. end result of successful adaptation
    B. relation between the person and his inner self
    C. relation between one's inner self and one's environment
    D. recognition of one's unconscious motivation (4:7)

47. The developmental history of an individual and of his illness is referred to as a/an

    A. abreaction
    B. anamnesis
    C. anamnestic reaction
    D. vita (4:11; 7:82)

48. Transsexualism is also known as

    A. transvestitism
    B. sex-role inversion
    C. bisexuality
    D. hermaphroditism (4:98)

49. Sexual identity is disturbed in the

    A. hermaphrodite
    B. homosexual
    C. pedophil
    D. all of the above (7:1411)

50. The conscious, predisposition to act is best defined as

    A. conation
    B. cognition
    C. affection
    D. reason (4:22; 7:345)

51. In Freudian theory, Thanatos refers to the opposite of

    A. anima
    B. libido
    C. Psyche
    D. Eros (4:26)

52. Depth psychology focuses on

    A. conscious mental processes and behaviors
    B. unconscious mental process
    C. mystical religious influences
    D. historic and anthropologic influences (4:29)

53. The therapy used by the psychobiologic school of psychiatry is called

    A. analytic psychology
    B. reality therapy
    C. behavioral therapy
    D. distributive analysis and synthesis (4:30)

54. Entropy accounts for decreased spontaneity for change in

    A. schizophrenics
    B. senescence
    C. psychotherapy
    D. adolescents (4:36)

55. The philosophic viewpoint of existential psychiatry is a

    A. culturally deterministic one
    B. holistic one
    C. biologically deterministic one
    D. all of the above (4:38)

56. Gender identity is a/an

    a. biologic concept
    b. cultural concept
    c. social expectation
    d. inborn response

    A. a only
    B. b and c
    C. a and b
    D. a, b, c, d   (4:41)

57. The "abstinence syndrome" suggests the presence of

    A. drug dependence
    B. addiction
    C. involuntary withdrawal
    D. all of the above   (4:6)

58. Psychoanalytically, pregenital refers to the

    a. oral phase
    b. anal phase
    c. latent phase
    d. pre-adolescent phase

    A. a only
    B. a and b
    C. a, b, and c
    D. a, b, c, and d   (4:75)

59. Psychoanalytically, the primal scene refers to an observation that is

    a. real
    b. fancied
    c. universal
    d. unconscious

    A. a only
    B. b only
    C. a and b
    D. a, b, c, d   (4:76)

60. The belief that one's thoughts can influence the throw of dice is

    A. parataxic distortion
    B. pychogenesis
    C. parapraxis
    D. psychokinesis   (4:78)

61. Satyriasis is analogous to

    A. frigidity
    B. impotency
    C. nymphomania
    D. onanism   (4:86)

62. A father says that his son shouldn't defy him, yet, he also complains that his son doesn't stand up to him like a man. This is an example of

    A. symbiosis
    B. mystification
    C. double-bind
    D. dereism   (20:317)

63. Hypermnesia is occasionally seen in

    a. dissociative reactions
    b. paranoia
    c. catatonia
    d. alcoholism

    A. a and d
    B. b and d
    C. b and c
    D. c and d   (20:119)

64. The phantom phenomenon is closely related to

    A. hallucinations
    B. delusions
    C. illusions
    D. obsessions   (20:102)

65. Confabulation is an example of

    A. hypermnesia
    B. amnesia
    C. paramnesia
    D. retrospective falsification   (20:120)

66. A person walks into a new restaurant and experiences the feeling that he has been there before. This is an example of

    A. jamais vu
    B. deja vu
    C. la belle indifference
    D. paramnesia   (20:121)

Directions: MATCH the following numbered items (role induction techniques), with the appropriate lettered item (neutralizing technique).

Questions 67 to 71

67. Coercing   (13:58)
68. Coaxing   (13:58)
69. Evaluating   (13:58)
70. Masking   (13:58)
71. Postponing   (13:58)

    A. Provoking
    B. Defiance
    C. Denial
    D. Refusal
    E. Disclosing

Directions: For each of the following multiple choice questions, select the ONE most appropriate answer.

72. Which of the following disorders is apt to be characterized by ego syntonic behavior?

    A. conversion reaction
    B. schizophrenia
    C. alcoholism
    D. depression   (10:204; 6:III:23–25)

73. The general adaptation syndrome (GAS) is a/an

    A. physiological response
    B. psychological response
    C. functional disorder
    D. organic disorder   (16:52)

74. The technique of talking about anything that comes to mind no matter how irrelevant it might initially seem is called

    A. perseveration
    B. free association
    C. loosening of association
    D. alliteration   (20:9)

75. All of the following statements about ego psychology are true *except* that it is

    A. in direct contradiction to Freudian theory
    B. an extention of Freudian theory
    C. concerned with the direct study of normal or healthy behavior
    D. concerned with the study of ego functions that develop from conflict and those that are conflict free   (1:3)

Directions: MATCH the numbered term with the letter of the most descriptive word or phrase.

Questions 76 to 82

76. Ontology   (12:253)
77. Amnesias   (12:236)
78. Syndromes   (12:233)
79. Reciprocal action   (12:244)
80. Transcendence   (12:253)
81. Gestalt   (12:245)
82. Cybernetics   (12:250)

    A. Interaction
    B. Feedback systems
    C. Configuration
    D. Analysis of being
    E. Groups of symptoms
    F. Ability to stand outside of oneself and observe oneself
    G. Memory gaps

C. Psychology and Literature

Directions: For each of the following multiple choice questions, select the ONE most appropriate answer.

83. The mother, as the son's love object, has been creatively described in which of the following literary works?

    a. *Tom Jones*
    b. *Desire Under the Elms*
    c. *Hamlet*
    d. *King's Row*

    A. a and d
    B. b and c
    C. a, b, and c
    D. a, b, c, and d   (21:114–15)

Directions: Match the following numbered literary works with the letter that describes the pathological state or diagnosis. Letters can be used more than once.

Questions 84 to 93

84. *Three Faces of Eve* (6:III:161)
85. *I Never Promised You a Rose Garden* (2:332–35)
86. *The Savage God* (32:19, 23)
87. *Lisa and David* (7:1356)
88. *A Child Called Noah* (6:II:89–90)
89. *The Bell Jar* (20:110–11)
90. *Lolita* (12:216–17)
91. *The Barretts of Wimpole Street* (20:412–19)
92. *Sybil* (20:81–2)
93. *The Caine Mutiny* (20:88–9)

    A. Paranoid personality
    B. Rhyming
    C. Infantile autism
    D. Multiple personality
    E. Depression
    F. Conversion hysteria
    G. Schizophrenia
    H. Suicide
    I. Drug addiction
    J. Pedophilia

Questions 94 to 103

94. *The Mingled Yarn* (20:315)
95. *Jordi* (6:II:89–90)
96. *The Story of O* (6:III:316–33)
97. *Hamlet* (21:115)
98. *A Moon for the Misbegotten* (11:10–17)
99. *Conundrum* (20:506)
100. *In Cold Blood* (6:III:258–62)
101. *Who's Afraid of Virginia Wolfe?* (21:334)
102. *Long Day's Journey Into Night* (20:512)
103. *Rebel Without a Cause* (6:III:255–58)

    A. Transexualism
    B. Pick's Disease
    C. Alcoholism
    D. Infantile autism
    E. Sadomasochism
    F. Unresolved Oedipus Complex
    G. Schizophrenic family
    H. Drug addiction
    I. Antisocial personality
    J. Conversion hysteria

Questions 104 to 111

104. *The Power and the Glory* (11:10–17)
105. *The Silver Cord* (21:115)
106. *Death of a Salesman* (18:163–66)
107. *Anna Karenina* (6:III:812)
108. *Summer Before the Dark* (18:170–72)
109. *Symbolic Realization* (20:332–34)
110. *The Painted Bird* (6:III:258–62)
111. *A Death in the Family* (32:10–12)

    A. Anaclitic relationship
    B. Narcissistic personality
    C. Antisocial personality
    D. Pedophilia
    E. Climacteric
    F. Normal mourning
    G. Unresolved Oedipus Complex
    H. Conversion hysteria
    I. Multiple personality
    J. Alcoholism

Chapter V: Answers and Explanations

1. **C.** Resistance to change increases in response to direct pressure for change. In this case, the staff nurses probably were defensive since they perceived the students' observations as criticisms of their behavior.

2. **B.** There is an almost universal tendency to seek to maintain the status quo on the part of those whose needs are being met by it. Therefore, even though personal contacts between the student nurses and staff nurses may be helpful in promoting increased understanding of roles and ideas and thus increased trust and may indeed help to sway a few pivotal staff nurses, the students need to be aware of the tremendous tendency for the staff nurses toward adhering to their own established group norms and behaviors.

3. **B.** Resistance to change based on fear of the new circumstances is decreased when those involved have the opportunity to experience the new ones under conditions of minimal threat. By focusing on one particular situation (narrowing the field), the students will have a better chance of succeeding than if they sought initial change by the staff nurses in many areas of patient care.

4. **D.** Although all of the statements are true, D is the answer that best guides the nurse's behavior. The law does recognize that, once aid is offered, it must be done properly and the assumed responsibility cannot be abandoned.

5. **C.** Nurses are specifically responsible to patients for improperly following orders or for following orders when they should have used independent judgment to the contrary.

6. **D.** Under nonemergency circumstances, the competent, conscious adult patient should be informed of the needed medical treatment and asked to give his permission in the form of written consent, if possible. However, the law recognizes several broad exceptions to the need for obtaining consent: the incompetent adult, the unconscious patient, the victim in crisis, and the individual openly assenting to treatment.

7. **D.** The Good Samaritan Law does not apply to situations in which a professional is called to an emergency in an official capacity or in response to a telephone call. It applies to the situation in which the professional comes upon an accident as a private citizen who also happens to be a crisis worker.

8. **D.** If a patient is unwilling to remain under care, the nurse has three alternatives. If he is a suicidal risk or so emotionally disturbed that he is incapable of protecting himself, he may be suitable for involuntary commitment. Likewise, if he is in life-threatening danger, he may be involuntarily committed. Otherwise the patient is permitted to sign himself out "against medical advice." If he refuses to do so, the nurse should carefully record that the patient has been warned of the serious potential danger to himself and that he refused to submit to care.

9. **A.** A hospital no longer has the right to turn away unwanted patients at the emergency room door. If a hospital holds itself out as offering emergency facilities, it owes an institutional duty of treatment to patients who seek its services. Moreover, this warrants the availability of competent staff, decent equipment, and reasonably attainable physician back-up.

10. **B.** The Good Samaritan law was adopted by almost all states because of a hesitancy on the part of professionals to render accident care on the scene for fear of possible lawsuit. In approximately one-half of the states, nurses are included in the statute.

11. **A.** It is essential that the emergency worker introduce himself by first telling the patient what he is: a physician, a nurse, a policeman, and then offering his first name as well as his surname.

12. **D.** If asked if other people are injured and the nurse knows, she should tell the victim. However, details should not be given. It is preferable not to report directly at this time to the victim that others have been killed. Words like "badly injured," "pretty bad" or "my partner is over there with them now" are better initial hedges at this point.

13. **D.** The emergency worker must be aware that he is in himself, an instrument of help. Awareness of and responsibility for the use of his body, whether it be to touch with his hands or his eyes or to talk, should be part of his repertoire. A victim's anxiety and fear can be appreciably minimized by appropriate talk, touch, and behavior.

14. **B.** A patient who *voluntarily* enters a psychiatric hospital retains all of his legal rights and civil liberties, including the right to be discharged from the hospital if he demands it. A driver's license is not a right, rather a privilege one earns by passing a test. Sometimes, patients on high doses of medication are under written doctor's orders not to drive a car.

15. **D.** Special consent on a printed form is required. The patient and his nearest relative sign the consent form. The law holds that consent must be based on an understanding of the treatment and its possible complications. The signed form should be on the chart before the treatment is given.

16. **D.** Currens Formula is a ruling that a person is not responsible for a crime if, as a consequence of a mental disorder, he did not have "adequate capacity to conform his conduct to the requirements of the law." The McNaghten Rule is a formula that holds a person not responsible for a crime if the accused "was laboring under such a defect of reason from disease of the mind as not to know the nature and quality of the act; or if he did know it, that he did not know he was doing what was wrong." The Durham Decision is a ruling which states that a person is not responsible for a crime if his act was the product of mental disease or defect.

17. **B.** The person must know that he is drawing up a legal document in which he is distributing his property in the event of his death. He must know the kinds of property he has and be able to remember by name, three persons to whom he might reasonably leave his property. He may have a psychiatric illness and still make a valid will if he fulfills these three criteria.

18. **C.** A voluntarily admitted patient who elopes from the hospital can be brought back only if he consents.

19. **B.** A voluntary commitment is to be distinguished from a "voluntary admission" in that in the former case, the hospital has the right to detain the patient for a legally defined period of time after he has given notice that he wishes to leave.

20. **C.** A patient who is committed by court action to a psychiatric hospital retains all his legal rights and liberties except the right to leave the hospital and terminate treatment without the permission of the psychiatrists who are caring for him.

21. **A.** The only states which have laws making nurse-patient relationships privileged are Arkansas, and in some cases, New York, New Mexico, and South Dakota.

22. **D.** An assumed role is one taken on in play or games.

23. **B.** An achieved role is one that is earned and involves effort and satisfaction of prerequisites.

24. **C.** An adopted role is informal and no permission is needed.

25. **A.** An ascribed role is universally expected; it usually includes age and sex roles.

26. **D.** It is assumed as it is done in a "pretend" sense.

27. **A.** Pattie is ascribed the role of a child due to her age.

28. **B.** An election indicates an achieved role.

29. **A.** This is an ascribed "sex" role of mother.

30. **D.** In role playing, a person acts "as if" he were someone else.

31. **C.** Thomas adopts the role of defender.

32. **B.** Psychiatry is the medical specialty devoted to the study and treatment of disordered feelings, thinking, and interpersonal relationships. Psychology and psychiatry merge at many points.

33. **B.** Cathexis is emotional investment in a person, object, or idea.

34. **A.** When we send a message either consciously or unconsciously, we also send a message about the message which is termed metacommunication.

35. **C.** Schizophrenia, the most severe functional disorder, is felt to arise from traumatic rejection during infancy. Manic-depressive psychosis has been associated with severe separation anxiety. The obsessive-compulsive reaction is seen as a result of trauma during the muscle-training period. Conversion reaction is seen as related to the Oedipal stage.

36. **C.** Goffman calls this, "civil inattention," an attempt between strangers to avoid one another's presence while forced to be physically close.

37. **C.** Ataraxy is the absence of anxiety or confusion—calmness. Thus, tranquilizers are frequently called "ataractic" drugs.

38. **C.** Apperception refers to the consciousness of the relation of new events, situations, or sensations to the individual's own emotions, past experiences, and memories.

39. **B.** Appersonification is the unconscious identification with another, sometimes famous person, in part or in whole.

40. **A.** The analytic rule in psychoanalysis is a rule for patients in therapy whereby the unedited and unselected voicing of free associations is undertaken in their order of occurrence.

41. **B.** Anankastia refers to any psychopathologic condition in which the individual feels forced to act, think, or feel against his will.

42. **B.** This effect was Cooley's construct and refers to the idea that we interpret what others think of us. It involves the following sequence: 1) the imagination of our appearance to others, 2) the imagination of their judgement, and 3) a self-feeling in response to this imagined judgement.

43. **D.** A system is frequently discussed in terms of morphostasis (structure maintaining) or morphogenesis (structure changing).

44. **A.** A placebo, in British usage called a "dummy", is an inactive substance originally given to "placate" a patient who demands medication that is not necessary. It has been found to be useful in research when double-blind studies are used.

45. **C.** The Hawthorne studies indicated that the highest motivation for the groups studied was neither money nor working conditions, but rather the fact that they were a special group being researched.

46. **A.** The end result of successful adaptation is termed adjustment. This consists of the relation between the person, his inner self, and his environment.

47. **B.** Anamnesis refers to the faculty of memory. It is information gained from the patient and others regarding his past medical history.

48. **B.** Transsexualism is also known as "sex-role inversion" and is believed to have its pathological origins in early childhood, when the future transsexual develops a primary and continuing identification with the parent of the opposite sex and adopts the gender role of that parent.

49. **A.** Sexual identity refers to the chromosomal condition, and to some extent, the internal genitalia which make a person biologically a male or female. This is to be differentiated from gender identity and gender role, which are psychological attributes.

50. **A.** Conation refers to the exertive power of the mind including the will and desire, as expressed in a conscious tendency to act.

51. **D.** Thanatos is the death instinct whereas Eros is the life instinct.

52. **B.** Depth psychology is the psychology of unconscious mental processes. It is also a system of psychology in which the study of such processes plays a major role, as in psychoanalysis.

53. **D.** Distributive analysis and synthesis entails extensive guided and directed investigation and analysis of the patient's entire past experience, stressing his assets and liabilities to make possible a constructive synthesis. It is the therapy of the psychobiologic school.

54. **B.** Entropy is the diminished capacity for spontaneous change such as occurs in aging.

55. **B.** In existential psychiatry, the philosophic point of view is a holistic and self-deterministic one. It focuses on the individual's subjective awareness of his style of existence, his intimate interaction with himself, his values, and his environment.

56. **B.** Gender identity denotes those aspects of appearance and behavior which society attributes to "masculinity" or "femininity." It is culturally determined, that is, what society expects.

57. **B.** The "abstinence syndrome" is equivalent to withdrawal symptoms and its appearance suggests the presence of physiological dependence or addiction. Drug dependence does not require physiological addiction. The syndrome occurs in both voluntary and involuntary withdrawal.

58. **B.** Pregenital refers to the period of early childhood before the genitals have begun to exert the predominant influence in the organization or patterning of sexual behavior.

59. **C.** In psychoanalytic theory, the primal scene refers to the real or fancied observation by the infant of parental or other heterosexual intercourse.

60. **D.** Psychokinesis is the belief that directed thought processes can influence an event.

61. **C.** Satyriasis is pathologic or exaggerated sexual drive or excitement in the male. Nymphomania is the analogous response in the female.

62. **C.** The father is giving two conflicting messages. Due to the intense emotional relationship with the parent, and the contradiction between the parent's verbal remarks and behavior, the son finds it impossible to discriminate properly. He can't ask for clarification since the questioning would be seen as a threat to the needed relationship.

63. **C.** Hypermnesia, abnormally pronounced memory, is occasionally seen in paranoia and catatonia. This excessive mnemonic capacity is largely limited to specific periods or events and experiences that are connected with particularly strong affects.

64. **A.** The phantom phenomenon or kinesthetic hallucination, is the hallucinatory perception of an amputated limb.

65. **C.** Paramesia, or falsification of memory, as well as distortion of memory, serves as protection against intolerable anxiety. In the form of confabulation, the patient fills the gaps in his memory by fabrication and accepts them as actual occurrences.

66. **B.** In this phenomenon, there is a feeling of familiarity on observing something of which there has been no previous observation, or of having previously lived through a current experience.

67. **B.** One person forces the other to accept roles by threats or punishment. It may be neutralized by defiance.

68. **D.** This involves the manipulation of rewards and may be neutralized by refusal.

69. **C.** Praising, blaming, shaming, approval, and disapproval are used. The specific neutralizing technique is denial.

70. **E.** Correct information is withheld or some other incorrect information is substituted. Unmasking or disclosing is the neutralizing element.

71. **A.** Time permits changes to take place that solve the conflict. Provoking is the neutralizing technique and incites the conflict to emerge.

72. **C.** The individual engaging in ego syntonic behavior does not experience it as painful, alien, or symptomatic. This is true of the chronic alcoholic.

73. **A.** Hans Selye describes three stages of physiological response to stress as the general adaptation syndrome.

74. **B.** The technique of free association was first used by Freud who found he had a means of exploring the earlier experiences upon which the patient's mental processes and current symptoms rested.

75. **A.** Although ego-analytic theorists agree that Freud has neglected the direct study of normal or healthy behavior, their work is an extension of Freudian theory rather than a contradiction of it.

76. **D.** Existentialism involves the analysis of being and focuses on the importance of human choice or decision.

77. **G.** The technique of free association in psychoanalysis leads to the uncovering of memory gaps which have arisen through repression of psychologically painful material.

78. **E.** Syndromes have been shown by longitudinal studies to be predictive of future symptoms or their absence.

79. **A.** Sullivan felt that human behavior is synonymous with interpersonal processes and that the interaction between two people defines the situation.

80. **F.** The existential therapist, rather than emphasizing the past, puts the emphasis on the future and what man can become, based on his own decisions and efforts. Man's ability to transcend or rise above the immediate situation is emphasized.

81. **C.** Gestalt is a German word meaning shape, form or characteristic entity. Gestalt psychologists point out that we do not perceive the environment as a mosaic of all its parts, but rather as a whole.

82. **B.** Cybernetics is that part of systems theory which deals with self-regulating or "feedback" systems.

83. **D.** The Oedipus theme has appeared in Fielding's *Tom Jones*, Bellamann's *King's Row*, Shakespeare's *Hamlet* and O'Neill's *Desire Under the Elms*.

84. **D.** The book by H. Thigpen and H. M. Cleckley is an example of multiple personality. The mechanism of dissociation is a means used by the ego for dealing with overwhelming anxiety.

85. **G.** Hannah Green describes the course of treatment of Deborah, a very disturbed schizophrenic young girl.

86. **H.** A. Alvarez describes his own unsuccessful suicide attempt at age 31, in the midst of a great precocious success as a critic.

87. **B.** Theodore Rubin's Lisa, uses the symptom of rhyming "Lisa's a girl, a pearl, a pearl of a girl."

88. **C.** Josh Greenfield writes of his autistic son.

89. **E.** Sylvia Plath describes a very depressed poet in a fictionalized autobiography.

90. **J.** Vladimir Nabokov describes a middle-aged man's infatuation with the 12-year-old Lolita.

91. **F.** Elizabeth Barrett Browning's conflict about her father's seductiveness and authoritarian overprotectiveness resulted in her being bedridden until she became engaged to Robert Browning.

92. **D.** *Sybil* is Flora Rheta Schreiber's case study of a girl with 13 different personalities.

93. **A.** Herman Wouk's, *Captain Queeg,* is a beautiful example of the paranoid personality.

94. **G.** Beulah Parker gives a vivid description of the interactions of a schizophrenic family.

95. **D.** Theodore Rubin's *Jordi* is the story of an autistic little boy.

96. **E.** Censured for many years, *The Story of O,* by Pauline Réage is a personal account of sadomasochistic behavior.

97. **F.** William Shakespeare deals with the unresolved Oedipal conflict in the young prince's ambivalence about avenging his father.

98. **C.** Eugene O'Neill writes of Jamie's struggle with alcohol in this well-known play.

99. **A.** Jan Morris tells of her early gender indentity problems and the change from the male, James to the female, Jan, following sexual surgery.

100. **I.** Truman Capote's chilling novel describes two characters, Richard Hickock and Perry Smith, both of whom are antisocial personalities.

101. **E.** Edward Albee's play offers a vivid example of a marital situation where both members of the couple derive gratification from both sadistic and masochistic behavior.

102. **H.** The mother in this classic play by Eugene O'Neill was a morphine addict.

103. **I.** Robert Lindner's book is a detailed example of a case report of a sociopathic or antisocial personality.

104. **J.** Graham Greene writes of a priest suffering from alcoholism in his novel.

105. **G.** Sidney Howard's play is the story of two brothers, sons of a seductive and possessive mother. One son, David, succeeds in breaking the bonds of childhood whereas the other brother never resolves his Oedipal attachment.

106. **E.** Arthur Miller's poignant story of a fading salesman in search of an identity emphasizes the crisis of the climacteric.

107. **B.** Tolstoy's heroine is a classic description of the progressive deterioration of one who lives in a narcissistic world of omnipotence.

108. **E.** Doris Lessing's novel recounts the "empty-nest syndrome" and the emergence of a middle age woman into her own being.

109. **A.** Marguerite Sechehaye's case study of the treatment of a severely regressed patient describes the process of anaclitic therapy.

110. **C.** Jerzy Kosenski writes of experiences after World War II that occur in the countryside of Europe.

111. **F.** This play by James Agee focuses on the effects of death on a family.